D0720437

THE 7 SYSTEMS OF BALANCE

The 7 Systems of Balance

A Natural Prescription for Healthy Living in a Hectic World

Paul J. Sorgi, M.D.

Health Communications, Inc.
Deerfield Beach, Florida

www.hci-online.com

Library of Congress Cataloging-in-Publication Data

Sorgi, Paul J.

The 7 systems of balance : a natural prescription for healthy living in a hectic world / Paul J. Sorgi.

p.   cm.

ISBN 1-55874-925-1 (tradepaper)

1. Quality of life. I. Title

BF637.C5 S65 2001

158.1—dc21

2001039272

©2001 Paul J. Sorgi, M.D.

ISBN 1-55874-925-X

Publisher: Health Communications, Inc.
3201 S.W. 15th Street
Deerfield Beach, FL 33442-8190

R-03-02

Cover design by Lisa Camp
Inside book design by Dawn Grove

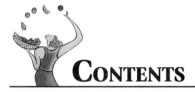

CONTENTS

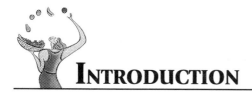

INTRODUCTION

> Bodily experiences, therefore, and more particularly brain experiences, must take place amongst those conditions of the mental life of which psychology need take account.
>
> William James (1842–1910) *The Principles of Psychology*

Are you feeling stressed? Are you tired, out of sorts, sleeping poorly? Do you feel overwhelmed by life? Are you nervous and uptight? Is your life out of balance?

If you read other self-help books about balance, you will no doubt be told that you must simplify your life to achieve balance: Cut down on your activities and commitments; work fewer hours; give up many of the possessions that you have worked so long to acquire; reduce your expectations. Then, and only then, after you strip your life of excitement, can you live a balanced life.

Hogwash!

Thanks to some breakthrough discoveries about the

workings of the brain and mind, it is possible to achieve balance in life while fully participating in a wide range of activities and interests. Researchers have clarified the rules for creating balance in life, which I will explain in this book.

In my work as a psychiatrist, I have helped thousands of people to heal the damage caused by today's hectic life, and in so doing, I have seen how balance can work. I will show you how you can make it work for you, by establishing a healthy balance in life through a program I call your "Rules for Living." The Rules for Living is a program of balance created from the natural workings of your brain and nervous system.

You will come to learn that you can live a life that is as full as you would like and still feel balanced. This is because balance comes from within the workings of your nervous system, not from the way that you set up your activity calendar.

What, you may ask, is the evidence for this? Science has proven it and so has my success with thousands of patients. The groundbreaking scientific discoveries, all of which have occurred within the past twenty years are as follows:

Brain Development

The brain systems that we use to live in our technologic society today developed as a result of the experiences of prehistoric, tribal humankind. While we live in a world of startling new technologies, we still function with a brain designed to understand and to live in a tribal, hunter-gatherer society. Furthermore, the very technologies we have created to make life easier, subtly unbalance the inner workings of our prehistoric, tribal nervous systems. Modern technology, in all of its wonderful abundance, helps us to live better lives. But at the same time, it also shakes and rattles our nervous system, which was created to respond to the cycles of nature and the rhythms of living with a small band of people. This book will show you how to realign your brain's activities to today's modern world.

The Seven Systems of Balance

The human brain is organized into discrete functional units that work as operating systems with a set of defined rules or instructions. These functional units can be thought of as "intelligences" or as operating systems. They are the seven systems of balance.

These discoveries come from the field of neuropsychology, a field that has exploded with knowledge in the past decade. Researchers have learned how to use specific neuropsychological tests to define these operating systems. From this work, it is possible to derive the "Rules for Living" that lead to balance.

This leads to a very different understanding of brain and mind function. Prior to this, you were either "smart" or "stupid." And the operation of your mind was ascribed to a vague notion of "character;" that is, you were responsible for the way your brain worked. It was a function of your willpower and discipline. After these discoveries, it has become clear that each person is born with very

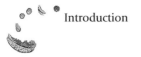

different brain systems which result in a different range of skills, abilities and operating rules. You can learn to manage the functioning of your brain by learning to use these operating rules. In doing so, you learn to better manage your life.

The Balance of Structure and Passion

The basic functional unit of each brain system is a balance circuit made up of an energy source, from the lower centers of the brain, and a cognitive (or thought-based) structure that takes the energy source and shapes and guides it into purposeful action. Powerful brain imaging tools can actually picture these brain circuits in action. From these pictures you can see the balance of energy (I call this energy, "passion") and structure in the brain's operating systems.

You can learn to influence the way that your brain balance circuits operate. You can learn how to infuse your day with the life energy that originates in your feeling brain. You can learn how to guide and structure your emotional life energy into rhythmic, flowing and purposeful action. And when you do, you will feel balanced.

While I don't profess that you will know in detail all of the inner workings of your brain at the completion of this book, you will learn how to balance your life by learning how to establish and maintain balance in your brain's operating systems. Balance comes from within. By understanding the intrinsic operating rules of your nervous system, you can live your life to the fullest while you maintain balance.

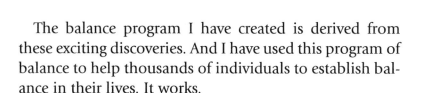

The balance program I have created is derived from these exciting discoveries. And I have used this program of balance to help thousands of individuals to establish balance in their lives. It works.

Now I want to share this program of balance with you. Come along with me on a journey of personal discovery. All you need is an open mind and a willingness to try.

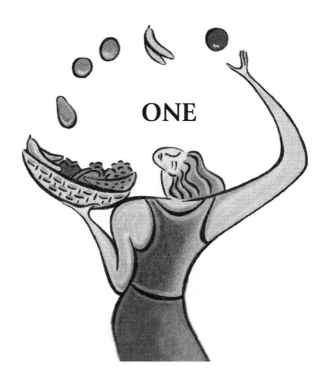

ONE

Why Is Life So Out of Balance?

Sometimes, on a plane at night, isolated from ordinary markers of time and place, you can get into a hopped-up, soaring mental state.

Nicholas Lemann, "The Word Lab," *The New Yorker*, October 16, 2000

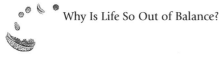

The Modern Problem of Balance

"I'm dealing with a possible divorce; my kids have been sick all week; I'm in debt. I have to work at night doing per diem nursing jobs to make ends meet. All I was really trying to do was to pursue my career as a nurse. I thought I had it all figured out. Then everything changed on me. It all sort of fell apart. I don't know what to do."

As a psychiatrist with over fifteen years of experience, I help many people like Kate. Does her story above sound familiar to you? Read on, and you will see why. This kind of problem is happening everywhere. Life presents you with exciting possibilities, you try to grab for the ring, to go for the challenge, and the next thing you know, you are up to your neck in troubles and stress.

What is it all about? We all live with ancient brains that developed over the past 7 million years. And modern life, with all of its wonderful technologies, presents our ancient brains with a type of stimulation and pace for which we are unprepared. Thus, your brain reacts as it did hundreds of thousands of years ago and you lose balance. The rules for living have changed. There is so much that is possible in your career, in your family, in your leisure time. Never before have people been able to do so much with their lives. But, as is the case with Kate, everyone also seems to be struggling with lives that are out of balance. Out of balance because the world has changed drastically in the last two hundred years, and there has not been enough time to develop new rules for living.

Let's return to Kate's predicament. It will help you understand what I mean.

If I could send Kate back to live in rural Ohio in 1800, her nervous system and her life would not be out of balance. The rules for living would be clear to her. She would know what to do. Kate would have close ties with about fifty people in her community. She would live with her extended family, either under the same roof or nearby. She and her parents, her brothers and sisters, her aunts and uncles and all of their children would gather each night around the hearth, to eat, to talk, to share stories, to comfort one another. If her marriage was failing, family and neighbors would step in to help. There would be no need to consider staying up late working because everyone went to sleep when it got dark. No one worked at night. There would be no struggle with job and family. She would take care of the kids full time. Of course that would include raising food, but the family would do that together. If they could not, then her friends and neighbors would tide her over until better times arrived. The rules to guide her behavior would be clear. The rules had been the same for thousands of years. Kate would know what to do.

Now fast forward to the year 2001. Kate's extended family lives thousands of miles away. She doesn't know all of her neighbors, and the ones she does know can't help her because they work all day. She wants to stay home with her kids but everyone tells her to get a job to support herself. So she stays up late working on her computer in her virtual office. Her husband is planning to move to Los Angeles and at the same time expects joint

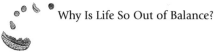

custody of the kids because "they can fly back and forth." There is not an hour of the day when her attention is not divided between kids, cell-phone calls, a television screen and her work. Kate's life is seriously out of balance. She feels miserable. She doesn't know what to do.

Consider all of the devices that we now have that were created in the past two hundred years. First came the industrial revolution, the automation of basic life-sustaining activities such as the production of food and clothing. In a matter of a few decades, food, clothing and shelter became widely available at low cost. Then came (in random order) the steam engine, electricity and electric lights, the automobile, the telephone, the airplane, the computer, the Internet, radio, television, cameras, video recorders, washing machines, microwaves.

Consider how life has changed. Dr. David Buss, writing in the *American Psychologist*, cuts right to the heart of the matter: "Modern environments have produced a variety of ills, many unanticipated and only now being discovered. . . . Modern humans . . . are bombarded by media images of attractive models on a scale that has no historical precedent and that may lead to unreasonable expectations. . . . Ancestral humans lived in extended kin networks, surrounded by genetic relatives such as uncles and aunts, nephews and nieces, cousins and grandparents. Modern humans typically live in isolated nuclear families often devoid of extended kin."

With all of the blessings that modern life bestows, consider the challenges it presents. Challenges that are so recent and profound that the impact on our well-being is barely understood.

What happens when you live apart from extended family, when there is no one to turn to for advice, or for help with the kids when you feel sick? What happens to you when your activity is not regulated by the natural rhythms of day and night, when you can watch television, work or socialize at any time of the day or night? What happens when you are bombarded by flickering video images no matter where you turn, images that change in a decidedly fast and nonhuman manner? What happens when you no longer need to get up, to move about or to do physical work for your food? What happens to you when you are just a number, a statistic, one of millions, helplessly buffeted about by an increasingly faceless and impersonal society? What happens when you can travel across great distances by airplane in just hours, landing in a completely new time zone, new climate and new culture? What happens when you no longer have to talk to others face to face, when you can transact human business by e-mail, cell phone, voice mail and fax?

All of this boggles the mind. Or, more to the point . . . it unbalances the mind and it can unbalance your life. It is no wonder that Kate is confused. Almost anything is possible in her life!

In my work as a psychiatrist, helping thousands of people, I have learned the secrets of balance. Through my research into the biologic principles of the nervous system, I have learned the secrets of balance. Come with me, and I will show you how balance works.

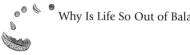

You will learn the first step to balance is passion because passion is the fuel that powers your brain and your life. Go after all that life offers. Make your life rich with reward and satisfaction. Be passionate about the people in your life, about your work, about the issues that really matter.

But passion alone is not enough. Passion is what got Kate into her fix. She had a passion for nursing that she pursued with vigor. She pursued her passion for nursing to the point that it caused an imbalance, in her marriage, in her family, in her health. It sure was exciting, but it caused so much disruption that her life fell apart.

Passion must be balanced with structure. Passion works best in the right place and in the right time. Then, like a finely tuned engine, all cylinders firing, all parts meshing and smoothly lubricated, your life will race ahead.

The secret to a balanced life is in the balance of passion and structure.

What does this have to do with modern life, you might ask? Quite a lot. The wonders of our age, all of the inventions, all of the new ways to do things, all of the new ways to be in contact with others, the access to any and all sources of information, all of the new ways to travel, all of these limitless opportunities make it possible for you to pursue your passion, your ideas, your interests, your love. Unlike any other time in history, you are not limited by your position in society. You are not limited by great distance between people. You are not limited in your access to key information. You are not limited by fear of disease or famine. It is the best of all times to be alive. Any person, from any walk of life, with the right combination of skill and hard work, can accomplish anything.

And so we do.

The trouble is that we have forgotten about balance. Limitless opportunity and possibility can lead to a frantic search for happiness. This is the modern dilemma. In pursuing our passion to be happy, we ultimately become unhappy. Why? The missing ingredient is balance. It is just how human beings are made. In order to be happy, your life must be balanced. Otherwise your body and brain send you powerful signals, telling you that something is wrong.

You see, your body and your brain are only trying to help you. The signals tell you that it is time to do something about the imbalance in your life or problems are sure to arise. If you think about it for a moment, it makes sense. Our bodies and brains developed during a time when life was dangerous. Our ancestors could easily go hungry, or get killed by a wild animal or a marauding band of humans, or they could easily contract a fatal disease. An imbalance was a sign of danger. Our ancestors only felt happy and at ease when all of their life-sustaining needs were satisfied. Only then, would they experience balance, the balance that came from having a full stomach, in a safe place, surrounded by family and friends. For the world of our ancestors, limitless possibility was dangerous. It meant you could starve, become ill or die a violent death.

In our world, limitless possibility is everywhere. Instead of being scared by it, we are energized (our ancestors were energized, too, but in their case, they were energized by fear). In our world, limitless possibility and pursuing passion is a good thing. It is what we all want. But our bodies and brains still react as if we are living in the world of our ancestors, 100,000 years ago. Our bodies and brains see limitless possibility and the pursuit of passion as a sign that danger is about.

The answer lies in balance. Pursuing passion is fine, so long as it is done with structure. Done in the right way, pursuing your passion can turn you on, it can lead you to new ground, it can help you to realize your dreams.

Let's return to the year 1800 to rural Ohio (I am focusing on rural life because even as long as two hundred years ago, city dwellers were already having balance problems). By this time, we human beings had figured out how to live a balanced life. But as you shall see, balance came at a cost. Modern life is better in a fundamental way, so long as you can maintain balance in your life.

In 1800 Kate would, in all likelihood, live her entire life within ten miles of home. She would live on or near the family farm. If her family was well-off, well positioned in society, then this would last throughout her life. If, on the other hand, her family was poor, there was no way for her to break the cycle of poverty. She would marry someone she had known since childhood; her husband may well have been a cousin. She would raise children and work on the farm. She would have a deep and stable involvement with her community and her church. She would become passionate about family matters—such as who was in good graces with the head of the family and who was on the outs, who was ill and who was healthy, who was in love and who was not—about local society, and about local politics. She would be passionate about survival, because in her world, survival was a key concern. Kate would spend hours worrying about and acting on outside threats, food supply and illness. These passions would be strongly balanced by the natural cycle of day and night—there were no electric lights—by the predictable routines of life, by the closeness of her family, by her strong community ties, by her sturdy religious beliefs and by the fact that her daily activities were unchanging. The balance in her life would be the same as the balance experienced by her ancestors for thousands of years in the past.

Kate's world in 1800 would be a world of conformity, of stable patterns and stable expectations. Possibilities were not limitless; they were, in fact quite limited. If she wanted a different life, she had only one choice, to leave home and become a pioneer on the frontier, endangering everything she knew and loved, just to change.

Thankfully, the modern age has given us the gift of practically unlimited possibilities for personal growth and change. And we can go after these challenges without being in danger. You can move or try a new career or even a new love life. You will not endanger your life or the life of your children by doing so. All that you risk is balance.

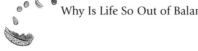

Modern Life Upsets Your Balance

Moore's Law, formulated in 1965, correctly predicts that the processing speed of computer chips will double every eighteen months. Today, desktop computers routinely perform tasks that room-size mainframe computers could not years ago. Computer games, e-mail, surfing the Internet are three common computer functions that were not possible twenty years ago.

During the Rennaisance, in the 1500s and 1600s, the printing press revolutionized the Western world. Then, it took several generations for this to occur. James Gleick, in his book *Faster*, describes the way it is today, when new creations move from conception to everyday life in an astonishingly short period of time.

"In the automobile industry, development cycles traditionally spanned five years. . . . By 1993 the cycle was down to thirty-nine months; by 1997, twenty-four months, but Toyota was boasting eighteen months and trying for fourteen."

A new car is created, moving from design ideas to the showroom floor in only twenty-four months! With computers, this cycle of creation is even quicker, with new computer designs reaching the marketplace in under one year.

We live in an age of wonders, unlike any other time in human history. New technologies, new medicines, new communication devices, new modes of travel, are created and produced at a dizzying pace. Just ten years ago, the Internet was only a gleam in the eye of some technology researchers. Now it is one of the most omnipresent and powerful forces in our society.

In today's world, if you have a dream, an idea or an inspiration, it can become a reality in just a few short years. The pace of technologic advance is so rapid, it is almost beyond human comprehension. Life, and what you can do with it, is changing so rapidly that it takes your breath away.

All of this directly impacts on human function: life-saving drugs; computer microchips to perform basic functions such as automated systems to fly airplanes, schedule your day, even cook your food; wireless communication tools like pagers, cell phones, even wireless fax machines to allow instant connection with others and to the world of information. These are new technologies that profoundly affect the way that we humans operate.

Think about the changes that just the combustion engine and the automobile alone have produced: suburbs, shopping malls, mega-industrial farms, commuting to work, even changes in sexual behavior (it can be argued that the rise in teenage sexuality is attributable to the independence that automobiles provide for teenagers).

New inventions, new technologies have extended our reach. Natural *human* limits, boundaries that separate what is possible from what is not, barely exist. Today, your life is filled with choices, with possibilities, with situations and circumstances that our grandparents could not have imagined.

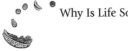
Living with Limitless Choice and Possibility

Your brain, your body and your nervous system are not new. Humankind has lived with the same brain chemicals, the same muscles, the same bones, the same instinctive reflexes and reactions for at least 500,000 years. If you believe in evolution, then the facts are more astounding. The same brain chemicals, neural signals and brain systems were present in our evolutionary ancestors over seven million years ago.

Delicately balanced brain systems developed as a result of circumstances that our ancestors confronted. Millions of years ago, this was an inescapable process. It was a brutal process, too. Our ancestors either developed in ways that helped them to survive or they died. The everyday challenges our ancestors faced were the struggle to find food and shelter; living through dangerous weather events, like drought; surviving the change of the seasons; fighting off aggressors and carnivorous animals; avoiding disease and injury; and, most importantly, the life and death challenge of having babies and raising children. The brain systems that made this possible developed over millions of years. These brain systems regulate sleep and energy level, eating, procreation, memory, planning, problem solving and social (or tribal) interactions. Our ancestors lived in balance because they had to—in those days it was a matter of survival.

Over 7 million years of life, these adaptations, the elements of balance became hard-wired into the brain.

Today, the life or death challenges that we humans face are, for most of us, a thing of the distant past. Yet each of us still functions today with a collection of reflexes, reactions and thoughts that are based on the lives that humans lived millions of years ago.

Imagine that. While our technologies change and develop each hour of the day, the human nervous system bumps along, unchanged in eons. That is where our modern problem with balance begins: *our ancient brains reacting to our modern inventions.* Brain systems that control and balance sleep, eating, sex, relationships, worry and planning, systems that are millions of years old, are unbalanced by the intrusion of our new technologies. Every day! No wonder it is so hard to maintain balance.

Look around. You will see balance problems everywhere. "Chill out! Juggling Too Many Tasks Takes a Toll, Researchers Say." This is a quote from the May 20, 2000 edition of *The Boston Globe.* The article goes on to say, "recent studies show that people can juggle a fair number of tasks. . . . But dividing their attention often makes them exhausted, stressed and forgetful." From the June 3, 1998 edition of the *Wall Street Journal,* "Teens Are Inheriting Parents' Tendencies Toward Work Overload." The *Wall Street Journal* article describes the problem, "One student, 16, . . . says, 'I'm over my limit. I'll stay up until 5 A.M. if I have to.' . . . Studies of teens . . . show that those who feel stressed by conflicting demands tend to drink too much and get depressed."

The collapse of the Soviet Union, and the subsequent modernization of Russia provide more signs of imbalance.

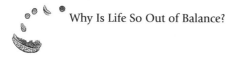

Research published in *The Journal of the American Medical Association*, in March, 1998, shows that as Russia modernized, as the Russian economy responded to market forces, as new technologies were introduced on a widespread basis, a social crisis has occurred. Life expectancy has plummeted; the Russian people are dying at a younger age. Why? Because there is a skyrocketing rate of alcohol abuse and of tobacco use. Because there is a dramatic increase in heart attack and strokes. Because there is a dramatic increase in deaths from suicide, homicide and automobile accidents. Why is this happening? Because the rapid pace of modernization is destroying the usual balance of the Russian people. Without balance, people suffer stress and stress-related problems.

Our problems with balance are so widespread that companies have been formed to make money from today's "out-of-balance" lifestyle! A new company, Urbanfetch.com, promises free delivery of over fifty thousand different items, that people "need" twenty-four hours per day. Urbanfetch.com promises to deliver items as diverse as ice cream or pizza, cold medicines, DVD players, even air conditioners, within one hour, no matter what time of day or night it is. And, people are using the service. Urbanfetch.com reports a brisk flow of orders, for all items throughout the night. No longer must people fetch their own food, do their own shopping, sleep at night, talk to people in stores (Urbanfetch.com is an Internet "store"). With Urbanfetch.com available at a price, people do not even need to get up from their desks! If you want, you can work away at your computer, twenty-four hours per day, while all of the necessities of life are delivered to you. All you must do is stop work for bathroom breaks, at least until someone develops a technology for efficiently eliminating human waste, while you work!

We have seven fundamental brain systems that nature hard-wired into our nervous systems over millions of years. These brain systems helped our ancestors get the right amount of sleep, to eat and procreate, to solve problems, to plan actions, to avoid danger, to move and rest in a healthy balance and to live together in villages or in tribal units. Our ancestors lived in balance with the natural structure imposed by their environment; they lived in balance with the natural limits imposed by the workings of their own bodies; they lived in balance with the natural structure and rhythms of day and night, of the seasons and of the circumstances of their life. There was really no choice, no other possibility.

Modern life upsets this balance. Of course it does! We are a creative and inventive species. Humankind has diligently worked to create new technologies that help us to overcome natural limitations. And, now we have. But since we function with an out-of-date nervous system, our brains have some trouble adjusting to all of the new technologies. We pursue our passions, all of the possibilities that modern life brings and then we lose our balance.

Here is an example of the way in which pursuing passion in our modern world leads to balance problems.

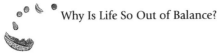

Her Family Is Happy, But She Isn't

Joanne is a beautiful woman with auburn hair, who always appears to be gazing off into the distance. At a time in her life when she should be enjoying the results of her years of hard work—her children are grown and on their own; her husband has a successful career; they are financially secure—at a time when she could be turning her attention to years of pleasurable activity with her family, Joanne's life is falling apart.

"All I ever really wanted was a happy family," she said sadly. "That's where all my energy went. I think that caused the problems."

"How can that be?" I asked. Joanne was beginning to look nervous. She was fidgeting with her purse.

"My husband says I'm a perfectionist and that all my worrying is making him nuts," she answered.

"What do you worry about?" I asked. It seemed like we were getting close. Joanne started to cry.

"Everything," she said in a flood of tears. "I'm sorry, it's just gotten so bad. At first, I worried about the kids. Were they sick, did I say the right thing to them, were their friends nice to them? Then it sort of grew. I worried that the house wasn't neat enough. I spent hours and hours cleaning. I worried that I was getting fat, so then I worried about what I ate. I worried that people would think our home was ugly and messy, so I stopped inviting people over. I started to worry about saying the wrong things in public, especially when I had to socialize with my husband around work. The craziest thing was that I began to worry that my husband was interested in someone at work. So I started to get on him about the amount of time he spent working and who he was with."

"It sounds terrible, like you felt out of control," I offered.

"I did. My solution was to spend more time alone, in bed reading. It was the only way I could stand it. I neglected everyone and everything but my kids and my home. It's awful. Now Ed wants a divorce. My kids are losing their patience with me. They don't even visit anymore. Who can blame them? I'm miserable to be with."

At one time, Joanne had worked as a nurse. Gradually, over the years, she stopped working to focus all of her energies on her home and her family. *"I wanted the perfect home,"* she told me. She went after it with a passion—the same passion that made her a superb nurse, energetic, creative and devoted to her patients.

The missing piece for Joanne was balance.

"At the end of my shift, when I was working in the intensive care unit, I usually felt pretty good about what I had accomplished. My patients were grateful. Nursing is really just people work, but I gave good nursing care, too. It was satisfying. When I left work, I figured I would get the same satisfaction from my home and my family. I did at the beginning. Until my worries took over."

Joanne was right in one way. Being a mother and a homemaker is an important job. It could have provided her with the kind of satisfaction that nursing did, if she had been able to achieve some balance. Instead, her natural high energy, her hard-working nature and the tendency she had to want everything to be perfect, caused her to lose her balance. Because she was able to do everything herself, she did. In doing so, she lost contact with people. Endless hours of cleaning; trip after trip to schools and to activities; hours and hours helping her kids with homework; shopping for food, clothing and all of the necessities

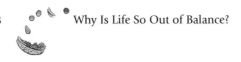
of modern life; she did it all. Friendships and social contacts drifted into the background. Missed lunch dates turned friendships into phone relationships. When the only time Joanne could find to communicate was late at night, her social contacts changed again, into distant e-mail relationships.

"Soap operas were my salvation," Joanne said, "the soaps gave me some contact with people, even if they are a little silly."

With her natural energy turned into worry over every detail, no longer certain of how to behave socially after years spent with her kids, Joanne spent any extra time she had alone, in bed with a book or in front of the television. Her life was completely out of balance. Her life was falling apart. She sacrificed her balance to pursue the passion she had for her home and family, and now she may lose it all.

The Secret to a Balanced Life

Here we are, living in a technologically advanced, modern world with an out-of-date nervous system. We all share in Kate's predicament. The world has changed so fast that our prehistoric nervous system has trouble keeping pace. If only life were simple. If only you could live in a village of two hundred people, living in an agrarian, subsistence economy. Then life would be balanced.

Who would want to do that? Not me. Not anybody I have met in the past fifteen years. Life today is fun. It is exciting, rewarding and full of interesting possibilities.

Instead of returning to a prehistoric village, consider that a life in balance is possible. In fact, your brain is set up to operate in balance. A natural balance is quite possible for you. This is exciting. Once you learn how to live with your own natural balance, the impossible becomes possible. You can go after your passion, live life to the fullest and live in balance.

Your brain balance systems are already hard-wired in place and ready to operate in a balanced way. The problem we all face is *not* that balance is hard to achieve. It isn't. The problem we all face is that modern life is so exciting, so interesting, so compelling, that it is just too easy to get carried away with it all and in doing so, you lose your balance. You can see this clearly in Joanne's story.

When you learn how to let your body and your brain do what comes naturally, you will live in balance. When you learn how to let yourself follow the natural rhythms of day and night you will live in balance. When you learn how to live with the natural rhythms of movement and rest you will live in balance. When you learn how to live with the natural rhythm and flow of your passions you will live in balance.

Why? *Because that is how we humans are made!*

Over the past forty years, careful research has uncovered the secret workings of the brain. Researchers have proven that your brain works best in balance. At all levels. From the way that two brain cells interact, all the way up to the level of behavior-controlling brain systems, your brain works best in balance.

The fundamental principle for your brain, the principle mentioned earlier in this chapter, is the balance between energy and thought. That is really how your brain works.

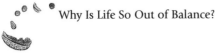

Instinctive mental energy balanced by conscious thought. At all levels. Really!

It is a practical system. All biologic systems are practical. Nature uses the materials at hand, in the most efficient way possible, to produce the needed effect. Your brain is a biologic system; underneath all of the fabulous thought, underneath the soaring creativity, underneath the passionate emotion, underneath what we think of as mind, is a physical organ—your brain—operating biologically, operating according to the rules of nature.

Energy balanced by thought. This is a fundamental natural rule of the way that biologic systems work. What does this mean? For your brain and mind, here is the translation. There is energy from older, lower centers of your brain that powers the nervous system, and there is thought from the newer, higher centers in your brain that modify and channel that energy, turning it into useful activity. This is a fundamental equation of nature. The equation can be described another way:

Energy + Thought = Purposeful, Balanced Activity

If you understand this basic equation, if you understand the way that the human nervous system developed to be in balance with prehistoric life, then you can begin to understand how to live in balance.

Passion is the key. Passion is the way that I refer to the energy from the lower centers of your brain. Passion could also be called psychic energy, emotion or drive. In natural balance, passion powers your brain, it is the fuel source for purposeful action. Passion works in balance with brain systems that modify and channel your passion into useful, purposeful and satisfying activity. Remember that these brain balance systems developed in response to prehistoric needs. Your brain balance systems developed in response to the cycles of day and night; in response to the cycles of birth and death in a primitive culture; in response to the pattern of life in a small tribe or village; in response to survival needs for food, shelter and protection.

Your brain balance systems did not develop in response to electric lights, telephones, automobiles, computers or television. With our wonderful inventiveness, we humans created these technologies long after our brain balance systems developed.

All that is required to live in balance is to let your passion, your brain's natural energy, work in balance with your higher-brain functions in the way that it did for our ancestors. All that is required is a program of balance, using some simple and commonsense steps, to recreate important elements of an environment that your brain balance systems understand. When you understand your passion, your energy source, you can learn how to use it to live in a productive balance. When you understand the way that your thinking brain naturally structures, inhibits, modifies and balances your passion, then you can learn to use these systems to produce a productive balance.

The secret to balance is that your brain balance systems work as though you still lived in prehistoric times. Fortunately, it is not necessary to live like our ancestors did to achieve balance. As I have said, who would want

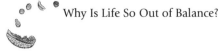

to? What *is* necessary is to learn how to live within the rules of balance for your nervous system; rules that were established long ago.

Understand that your brain is deeply influenced by the cycles of day and night; understand that your brain is deeply influenced by how you move about; understand that your brain is deeply influenced by how many people you interact with each day; understand that your brain is deeply influenced by survival needs. If you do, then you can live in balance. And, if you do, then you can comfortably and happily get more out of your life.

Why Is Balance So Important to Me?

Maintaining balance has been a struggle for me throughout my life. My balance problems became critical when I started on the path to becoming a doctor. In medical school, I had to study and attend classes as much as sixteen hours per day. There was no time for anything else. As an intern and resident, there was so much work, so many night calls, that I became sleep deprived and lonely. Meaningful relationships withered. Friends drifted away—when my closest friends had children, I was in the hospital taking care of my patients; I didn't have time to visit my friends or to make it to their children's christenings. My first marriage ended in divorce. I had no time for my wife and no room in my emotional life for love— whenever we had time alone, my pager beeped, calling me back to my job.

The balance problems that filled my life did not stop when I finished training. The life of a practicing physician is one of the most out-of-balance lives you can imagine. My life certainly is. My life is filled with telephone calls, beeping pagers and medical records. As a physician, I am sedentary much of the time. There is often no time for meals or for relaxation. When someone needs my help, I respond.

My life as a doctor is fairly typical of the lives lived by my physician colleagues. Despite our dedication to promoting health and healthy behavior, we physicians, all too often, are examples of unhealthy, out-of-balance lives. That may be why there are higher than expected rates of alcoholism, divorce and suicide among physicians. That may be why disability claims filed by physicians have skyrocketed in the last decade. As our profession becomes more and more technologically oriented and less centered on people, physician's lives become increasingly out of balance.

I am not complaining. It is a wonderful life, one that I dreamed about and that I worked hard to accomplish. It is filled with rewards and satisfaction. But, it is only sustainable when I take active steps toward maintaining my balance.

As a psychiatrist, I have studied the secrets of the brain for twenty years. As I work with my patients every day, I see how the various brain systems that researchers have described affect the lives and functioning of the people that I treat. As I try to sustain my life as a physician, I have learned to apply the principles of balance to myself. It has helped. By using a program of balance, a program that I will explain for you in this book, I can push for all of the excitement, all of the satisfaction, all of the possibility that life today has to offer.

I call my program of balance my "rules for living." The rules are simple things that I try to do every day. The rules are based on what works best for me. My rules for living help me and my brain to function in balance.

Yet, my rules for living are not casual or circumstantial. Instead, my rules for living are personal operating principles that are based on the way that my brain works best. It is a program derived from my own natural balance. That is the secret to balance, following a program that is based on your own balance points; a program that is based on the balance of your own brain systems.

Reaching your dreams is all about natural balance. It has been for me. It can be for you. Read on and find out how!

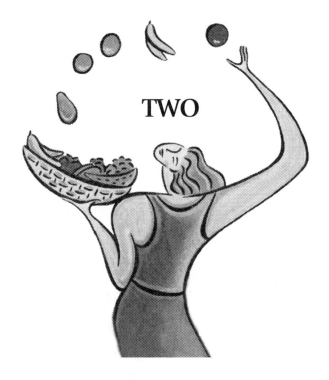

How Does Your Brain Work?

People are *born* resourceful and they *become* skillful and "thoughtful" when they genuinely care about what they are doing. One begins to understand the origins—and learns to appreciate the interdependence—of human skill, intelligence, and vitality by looking at the details, one piece and one person at a time.

Frank R. Wilson, *The Hand*

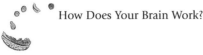

What Happens When
You Are Out of Balance?

There is no need to retreat from modern life; you do not have to live the simple life of our prehistoric ancestors. But to live a life filled with the possibilities and passion of today, you must do so with balance. That is our modern dilemma. Life these days just does not work harmoniously with our ancient brains. Life these days—as we live with all of the technologic advances that have freed us from the burdens of the past—filled with problems of balance.

Many of the life problems that trouble you are caused by balance problems. Many of your physical aches and pains are caused by balance problems. Many of your emotional concerns—the hurts and dissatisfaction that you try to shrug off and ignore—are caused by balance problems. Many of the problems and issues that you accept as part of life today, problems and issues that rob you of happiness, are a result of balance problems. When you know what to look for, you can see it everywhere: in yourself, in those you love, in your friends and in your neighbors.

But when your life is in balance, when you are functioning with a natural balance, then you feel well. A balanced life produces a sense of well-being. A balanced life allows you to feel happy, secure and satisfied. A balanced life allows you to feel rested and relaxed. A balanced life is a comfortable life with people you care about and who care about you. A balanced life feels healthy, and it is healthy. Researchers have shown that living in balance leads to a longer, healthier life.

When you are living out of balance, life just won't feel right—balance problems in your life can interfere with the natural, balanced functioning of your brain. All of the energy and excitement of modern life, has a way of getting right to the older parts of your brain, turning them on, triggering instinctive energy that leaves you feeling stressed, nervous and out of balance. You see, in the way that your brain is wired, these older parts of your brain, the lower centers of your brain, all take care of your physical needs. This part of the brain is dedicated to your survival. Naturally enough, since survival is the issue, your brain was created so that these circuits are the fastest, strongest, most automatic circuits in your nervous system. It is nature's way of trying to guarantee your survival. Your brain is wired to react to the facts of life for prehistoric man; any sign of balance problems in life is interpreted by your brain as a sign of danger.

The brain equation for the older, instinctive, lower centers of your brain is quite different than the equation for your complete brain in balance. You may recall the equation for your brain in balance is

Energy + Thought = Purposeful Action

For the older part of your brain, the equation is quicker, faster, a more direct route to survival based action. It is:

Energy = Protective Action

In the scenario that the older part of your brain understands, there is no conscious and rational thought channeling mental energy into purposeful action. The older

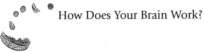

part of your brain senses and reacts with energy, not to establish balance, but instead to protect you from danger.

If you keep this scenario in mind, it becomes easier to understand and interpret the distress you may feel when your life is not in balance. Modern life is filled with constant change, constant stimulation coming at you with a frequency and intensity that is guaranteed to excite the instinctive energies of the older, lower parts of your brain. Your ancient brain reacts as it must, with an automatic outpouring of energy. Your brain reacts to modern life as though your village was about to be flattened by a tornado or attacked by a marauding band of hostile strangers. You become energized, alarmed and ready for danger. So, you spend much of your time out of balance, in a state of mind where your brain is alerting you to danger—even when there is none. You may be primed and ready to look for trouble, to react as if survival were an issue, when it is not. In fact, the opposite is true. And despite the always-present realities of crime and war—inherent in any society—this is the safest, healthiest, most secure time in history. What a paradox!

The trouble is that when the excitement, the challenge, the newness of modern life causes you to be out of balance, to live in survival mode, the result can feel terrible. In our prehistoric village, if you felt out of balance, it was time to take action, to do something to set matters right. In modern life, if you feel out of balance, there is nothing to set right! There is no danger lurking at the edge of your village; there is no threat to your survival for you to focus on. Modern life can cause you to feel wound up, nervous, looking for danger, with too much instinctive energy pouring out from the older parts of your brain. You can end up living this way for extended periods of time, which can cause problems. Month after month, year after year, living out of balance and in survival mode overtaxes your system and you burn out.

When your life is not in balance, when your brain is unable to function with a natural balance, when your older, instinctive brain systems all react with excess nervous energy, as if your survival were an issue, then you can have many of the following symptoms:

- unhappiness
- dissatisfaction
- excess worry
- trouble sleeping or inadequate sleep
- a constant sense of tiredness
- muscle aches, pains and stiffness
- overeating, overdrinking and overspending
- compulsive sex or no interest in sex
- excess nervousness
- edginess or feeling wired
- impatience
- uneasiness or feeling that something is about to go wrong
- being overly emotional
- low motivation
- lack of enjoyment
- boredom
- lack of confidence

- a sense of failure
- fearfulness

If you do have these problems, if you suffer with these symptoms, in all likelihood your life is out of balance and your brain is simply trying to tell you so. If that is the case, it is time to take action. It is time to restore balance in your life.

How Does Your Brain Function in Balance?

Excitation and stimulation, the energies that power the operation of your brain, come from the lower centers of your brain. These lower brain centers are called the brain stem, the subcortex and the limbic system. This ancient part of the brain generates the energy necessary for you to survive. It is somewhat like the power plant of the brain. It is the source of your emotions, your physical energy, your appetites and your survival instincts. This part of the brain, also present in animals, operates in balance with the circumstances of life, but only for the purposes of guaranteeing survival. It does not, and it cannot operate in a social balance. Creatures that live with only this degree of brain development live in isolation, concerned with eating, hunting, protecting themselves and procreating (at least at the right time). Mountain lions are an example of this type of animal. They are not social creatures. They live to survive, and they survive to live.

The lower centers of your brain work somewhat automatically. Usually, you do not have any conscious control over their operations. (You will notice that I said *usually*. It is possible to gain conscious control over the lower centers of your brain as part of a program of balance.) Usually you are not aware of the workings of the lower centers of your brain.

The modification and channeling of your mental energy into productive activity is the job of the higher centers of your brain. These centers are all located in your thinking brain, the part that scientists call the neocortex (this means "new cortex"). Researchers believe that these centers developed over the past 500,000 years, in response to the special needs that arose from social activity: from cooperation among individuals for the mutual benefit of all concerned. These centers control planning, memory, social interaction, higher reasoning, logic and deeply held beliefs.

You are aware of the activity of the higher centers of your brain. You perceive the activity as thought and as memory. Ordinarily, you can speak about your thoughts. You can describe what you are thinking. You know that you are using your intellect.

Thought, reason and belief can sometimes seem to exist apart from the workings of the rest of your brain. This can lead to the erroneous idea that mind is separate from body, that intellect is separate from emotion. This idea has existed for thousands of years, from Platonic idealism to the dualism of Descartes. This idea evolved from the simple fact that your lower-brain centers operate

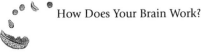
without the benefit of conscious thought and language, while your higher-brain centers, your intellect, operate almost exclusively with the biologic tools of conscious thought.

What modern life has proven, over and over again, is that when intellect is detached from emotion, when the higher centers of your brain are not operating in a natural balance with the lower centers of your brain, then you lose balance in your life.

The actual biologic facts are that the lower centers of your brain work in balance with the higher centers of your brain to produce satisfying, purposeful activity through a balanced process of energy and thought. Your lower-brain centers provide the energy and your higher-brain centers provide the thought, the structure to turn brute survival instincts into purposeful, meaningful human activity.

Putting this another way, your intellect, the higher centers of your brain, works best when charged with positive energy from the lower centers in your brain—when passion lights up your neocortex and sharpens your mind like a sunrise that lights up the day with bright pinks, blues and yellows. If you understand this, then you understand the basics of how your brain functions best.

Let's work with this idea a little bit, to get a better feel for it. The older part of the brain acts somewhat like the engine of a car. The engine of the car burns fuel and creates the energy needed to put the car into motion. The newer part of the brain is like the driver of that car. The driver takes all of that latent energy and pent-up motion, turning it into purposeful activity, like driving to the grocery store. (Your body would be like the body of the car: the fenders, the seats, the wheels etc.) The car could move without a driver. However, if it did, the movement would be undirected and dangerous. A driverless car, moving down the road, is certainly using the energy created by the engine, but to what end? The likely outcome is an accident! When you add the driver, you take all of the energy of the car and you *structure* it into a planned or purposeful trip. Now consider the opposite—a driver sitting in a car with no engine. What do you have? Well, you don't have useful activity. The driver will no doubt be planning a trip, but he or she will never go anywhere. Without the engine, all the driver can do is sit in one place, planning and thinking about going somewhere without actually moving. After a while, the driver would, in all likelihood, become upset with the whole enterprise, perhaps even somewhat depressed. There must be a balance between the engine of the car and the driver of the car. Then and only then can you get a purposeful, satisfying automobile trip.

The anatomy of the brain demonstrates this principle of balance, too. The lower centers of the brain, present in most complicated living creatures, come first. They are deep in the brain, closer to the vital processes necessary for life. The older part of the brain sits inside the newer part of the brain. The newer part of the brain, the neocortex, sits on top of the lower centers, the older centers of the brain. The neocortex literally surrounds the subcortex, the limbic system and the brain stem. To imagine how this looks, think of putting your hand in a mitten.

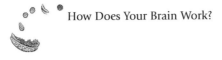

Then make a fist. Your fist is like the older part of the brain. The mitten wrapped around your fist is like the newer part of the brain, the neocortex, wrapped around the older parts of your brain.

This anatomic arrangement has a purpose. The newer part of the brain surrounds the older part of the brain because it structures, inhibits and controls the outpouring of life energy from the lower centers of the brain. The brain is structured so that the life energy from the lower centers of the brain must go through and be processed by the higher centers of the brain.

To bring this all back to the facts of day-to-day life, consider that your life will feel balanced when there is a natural balance between the older parts of your brain and the newer parts of your brain—a natural balance between the outpouring of life energy from the instinctive parts of your brain and the modifying influence of conscious thought. When there is a problem of balance, when modern life breaks the natural balance between your lower brain centers and your higher brain centers, then you feel it. You can feel the balance problem as stress. You can feel the balance problem as physical aches and pains or as sleep problems. You can feel the balance problem as an uptight nervousness, as trouble relaxing. You can feel the balance problem as a lack of patience, a tendency to anger too easily, a tendency to be too aggressive in your interactions with people. You can feel the balance problem in the way that it is difficult to control your eating, your drinking or your sexual activity. Most importantly, you can feel the balance problem as unhappiness. When you are out of balance, life just does not seem happy, fulfilling or satisfying.

What Makes Us Human

According to fossil records, human brain size increased dramatically between 1 million and 500,000 years ago. Why this happened is a subject of intensely interesting academic debate. The answer is still missing.

What is clear about this period of brain development, is that the part of the brain that expanded, the frontal lobes and the neocortex, is what makes us human. Behaviors that separate us from all of the rest of the living creatures on the planet—our human behaviors—are all produced by this part of the brain, the neocortex; specifically, the frontal lobes.

Each of the uniquely human balance systems came into being during this epoch. Each of these balance systems provides us with a piece of behavioral functioning that makes us distinctly, irreversibly and wonderfully human.

Here is a list of the brain behaviors that the higher brain centers contribute to balance:

- Planning and goal-directed behavior
- Learning from experience, memories of past events, patience
- Verbal reasoning and logic
- Social reasoning and interpersonal skills
- Belief in a stable set of values, spirituality or morality

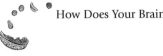
Each of these brain functions matches up with a particular lower brain function. The lower brain provides the power, the energy and the passion. The higher brain center provides the way to channel that energy into productive human behavior. The table below shows you the pairings, along with the balance system produced by that pairing.

Higher Brain Function	Lower Brain Function	Balance System
Planning and goal-directed behavior	Appetites for sex, eating, consuming	Appetites and abstinence
Learning from experience, memories of past events, patience	Drive to action, impulsivity, spontaneous reaction	Past and present
Verbal reasoning, logic	Reward, excitement and passionate interest	Thinking and feeling
Social reasoning, interpersonal skill	Fear and vigilance	Being alone and being with people
Belief in a stable set of values, spirituality, morality	Fear, worry and anxiety, avoiding danger and harm	Belief and doubt

Balance. Body and mind; energy and thought; linked together in a harmonious and rhythmic flow. The action of your thinking brain; thought, language, social understanding, images and visual relationships; is a structure or a channel for the social expression of your life energy. Each different type of thought works in a rhythmic harmony with a specific instinctive energy.

Systems of balance that make us human. That is the gift of creation. As humans, we can channel and structure our instinctive energies into planned and purposeful behaviors that allow us to be social beings; who care, who feel, who think, who count on one another.

That is the meaning of balance. Using the gift of thought in balance with the energies of life, producing a harmonious balance for ourselves and for those we care about.

Natural rules for balance flow directly from the brain systems outlined above. You will see these rules, you will learn your prescription for balance as you read through this book. Rules that guide you to a dynamic balance of energy and thought; rules that help you to stay balanced while you live with the excitement and passion of today; rules that work because they are based in the biology of your brain; your prescription for balance is created by your brain balance systems. Your natural rules for balance come directly from the way that your brain systems naturally balance energy and thought. For we social humans, living in groups, caring for each other, it is the way it has always been. Now more than ever, as modern life fractures traditional human bonds while creating new opportunities for living, it is essential to understand the dynamic flow of energy and thought. It is essential to understand how your brain was created to function in balance.

Controlling the Flow of Your Energy

For every creature on the Earth, with the notable exception of we human beings, the amount of time spent sleeping and the amount of time spent in physical activity is completely in balance with nature. The cycle of day and night and the rhythm of the seasons sets the timing and length of the sleep cycle. Survival needs determine the amount of physical activity that is necessary for life. These two essential bodily functions, sleep and movement, are naturally balanced by the circumstances of life.

That is not true for human beings. Through our wonderful inventiveness, we have unlinked sleep and movement from the structure of nature. The amount that you sleep, the amount that you physically move about is completely up to you! We have freed ourselves from the burdens imposed by nature. But, in doing so, we have also lost the natural and automatic way that these two key functions, sleep and movement, were balanced by nature. And so, in considering how to balance your life, unlike any other creature on Earth, we must learn how to balance sleep and how to balance movement.

With freedom comes responsibility. With freedom from the burdens of nature, comes the responsibility and the necessity for us to balance sleep and movement. What was once an automatic function, is now a fact of life. A modern responsibility, if you will.

Movement and sleep. Quite different from the social- and information-based balance systems of the frontal lobe. Yet, because movement and sleep control the flow of energy in your body and mind, taking care of your body by having a healthy balance of movement and sleep, is a requisite part of a prescription for balance.

Movement

In the distant past, at the very dawn of humanity, movement was thought. There was not a thought that was separate from movement. In the prehistoric past, thinking was only present to help coordinate and control movement. Movement was the substance of thought; mental representations of movement were our primitive language; movement patterns in the brain were the symbols used to think.

As a result, movement is inextricably linked to thought. Movement pathways are the pathways of thought. Mechanisms for controlling the flow of movement also control the flow of thought. Within the language and grammar of the brain, movement is the music of thought. Movement helps you process thinking and feeling in a flowing and harmonious rhythm. That is one reason why the absence of movement in modern life leads to problems of balance, because the lack of movement interferes with the way that your brain most efficiently processes thinking and feeling.

Movement is controlled automatically by the cycling of the cells in your movement centers. Your movement centers are located deep within the brain, in a central spot where your movement centers constantly communicate

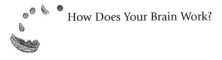
with all other parts of your brain. Your movement centers control the flow of movement and information through the action of two sets of cells operating in a reciprocal balance.

One set of cells secretes the chemical dopamine. When these cells are active, they squirt dopamine into your nervous system, telling your nerves and then your muscles to be active, to move and to think. But, the signal sent by the dopamine cells is wild and jerky. Alone, the message from the dopamine cells produces an uncoordinated, thrusting pattern of movement. These uncoordinated movements are modified into smooth and purposeful motion through balance provided by the other set of cells. These cells use the chemical acetylcholine. These cells counteract or inhibit the activity of dopamine (the motion chemical). The message that the acetylcholine cells sends is to stop: Stop moving, stop thinking, freeze up and wait. When the acetylcholine cells ("the stop cells") work alone, you become frozen, unable to move or think.

When the motion cells work in balance with the stop cells, then neurological magic happens. When these cells function in a balance of excitation and inhibition, you then have smooth, fluid, purposeful movement and thought.

Your movement centers function automatically to help you move smoothly, fluidly and effectively. Your movement center also works like a traffic cop, directing the flow of activity throughout the brain. Movement and brain processing activity are one and the same.

If you have a healthy amount of movement in your life then your movement centers are able to perform their job automatically. Remember, these brain centers developed to work for our prehistoric ancestors when movement was necessary for life. Your movement centers will work best when the amount of movement and exercise is far higher than it normally is for we modern humans; when the balance of movement and rest is more like it was for our ancestors.

With the proper balance of movement and rest in your life, then your movement centers function in an automatic and natural balance. A healthy pattern of movement in your life helps your brain, through the actions of the movement centers, to direct the timing and flow of thought, feeling and mental energy. Movement provides a script for balance. Movement provides music for the music of your mind; a graceful melody, the proper rhythm all coming together in a beautiful song.

If, like most people these days, you do not have enough healthy movement, then it is much harder for the lower centers of your brain to work in balance with your higher centers. Without enough movement, it is difficult to smoothly link energy and thought into meaningful and purposeful action. If you do not have a healthy balance of movement and thought, your mental efficiency and your sense of well-being suffer the consequences.

But if you follow some simple, natural rules for the balance of movement and rest, then energy and thought will flow in a fluid and harmonious rhythm. Natural rules about movement are natural rules about controlling the flow of your thoughts, your feeling and your mental energy.

Sleep

The energy of your mind is created by sleep. In a natural rhythm with the cycling of day and night, in natural rhythm with the cycling of the seasons, sleep creates energy for your mind. It is essential for balance. This is an obvious point, but one worth stating. Sleeping well, sleeping in a natural balance with your needs and with the natural cycles of the environment, creates energy for your mind. You need healthy energy to live in balance.

Sleep is controlled and regulated unconsciously by the cycling of the cells in your sleep centers. Deep in the center of your brain, in an area called the pons, are two collections of nerve cells. One set of cells secretes a chemical called norepinephrine. These cells and this chemical turn your brain on; when these cells are actively squirting norepinephrine into your brain, you become alert and energized. You wake up.

These alert cells are balanced by a set of cells that secrete a chemical called acetylcholine. These cells turn the awake cells off. When these acetylcholine cells do this, you sleep. When your sleep cells stop inhibiting your norepinephrine cells (your awake cells), then you wake up.

The awake cells and the sleep cells in your brain work in a natural balance. Your awake cells stimulate or excite all levels of your brain into an alert state; your sleep cells inhibit the awake cells, allowing you to get needed sleep. When working in balance, you sleep the right amount for your physical needs, and you are awake, alert and refreshed for the right length of time, given your physical needs. When you take sleep medication, you induce sleep by inhibiting your awake cells. A sleeping pill helps your sleep cells to work. When you take a stimulant, like coffee or caffeine pills, for instance, to help you to be alert, what you are really doing is helping your awake cells to work better, to be more excited and to escape the natural, balanced inhibition of your sleep cells.

Sleep balance is your energy balance. You cycle in and out of sleep as a way of recharging your batteries, physically and mentally. With the proper sleep balance, your brain and mind are refreshed and energized. It should all happen automatically. But as we will see in the next chapters, modern life is so stimulating, so captivating, in some ways it is so disturbing, that you lose the natural rhythmic cycle of sleep. You can quickly lose your natural sleep balance. The result can be an energy problem for your brain, for your body and for your mind.

When you are in a natural balance you can sleep. And when you sleep, you are able to live with a natural balance.

Is Balance Possible?

By this point in the book, do you find yourself wondering whether it is possible to make it all work, to live a balanced life?

Remember, our brain balance systems developed in our ancestors, over millions of years. Although your brain is more complicated than you can imagine, balance is not. The steps that you will need to follow to achieve a natural

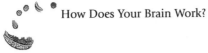

balance are simple and attainable. Your life probably has many of the elements of natural balance already in place. All you really need to do is emphasize some activities and deemphasize others. The following chapters will show you how.

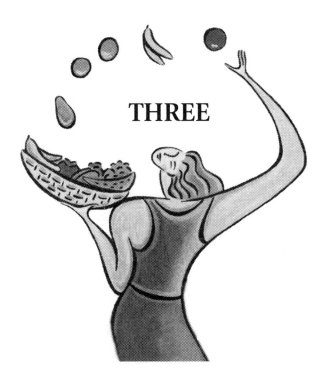

THREE

System 1:
Being Alone and
Being with People

While misery may love company elsewhere,
sardinelike proximity to strangers on trains and
buses kindles an assortment of antisocial feelings
from aggressiveness to indifference.

Winifred Gallagher, *The Power of Place*

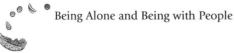

Too Much Togetherness?

Sometimes when you are surrounded by people, you are really alone. That is our modern dilemma. In perfecting ways to communicate, we have created technologies that we don't really know how to use. Sure, it is easy to understand what buttons to push, how to use America Online, how to use Direct TV to gain unlimited access to movies and television shows. The technology part is easy. The hard part is to figure out how our revolutionary technologies impact on our ancient brains. The hard part is to learn how to balance our modern-day informed and stimulated aloneness with our ancient need for people. Because as human beings, we have an ancient need for human contact that is sincere, that has a depth of emotion, that operates in harmony with who we are. Human contact that is uniquely suited to who we are.

Let's examine the problem. Here is a telling quote from David Shenk, in his book *Data Smog.*

> The blank spaces and silent moments in life are fast disappearing. Mostly because we have asked for it, media is everywhere. Televisions, telephones, radios, message beepers, and an assortment of other modern communication and navigational aids are now as ubiquitous as roads and tennis shoes—anywhere humans can go, all forms of media now follow: onto trains, planes, automobiles, into hotel bathrooms, along jogging paths and mountain trails, on bikes and boats . . .

Contact with people is the purpose for all of these

inventions. No matter where you go, no matter what you are doing, you are likely to be flooded with the words and pictures, voices and images of people. And that is just for communication devices.

Many of our inventions—inventions that are so much a part of life that we take them for granted—serve to bring you in direct contact with people; contact in a superficial, but nonetheless stimulating way. Elevators put you directly in close physical contact with a group of people you don't know. So do subways, buses, airplanes, shopping malls and sports arenas. Some almost invisible technologies, like electricity, advanced building design and climate-control technologies, allow you to live and work in close contact with thousands of people every day—in cities and in high-rise buildings.

Consider some facts that provide a picture of how we are flooded with contact every day.

- In 1971, the average American was targeted by at least 560 daily advertising messages. Twenty years later, that number had risen sixfold, to 3,000 messages per day.
- Telemarketing companies are one of the best examples of the superficial contacts generated by technology. More than 1,000 telemarketing companies employ 4 million Americans and generate $650 billion in annual sales.

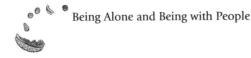

- Executives at high-tech companies now receive 150 to 200 e-mail messages per day. That is 20 to 30 per hour for an eight-hour day.
- In 1850, 2 percent of the world's population lived in metropolitan areas of 100,000 or more; by the year 2000, 40 percent did.
- Over 90 percent of U.S. households have color televisions. Over 80 percent have VCRs.
- In five years, Americans purchased 85 million color televisions, 48 million VCRs and 23 million cordless telephones.

Although we live in a time of unparalleled connection, it is also a time of confusion. Signs of widespread balance problems in our contact with people are emerging. Disconnection, rudeness and a lack of common decency are becoming an epidemic. We are so overstimulated with human contact that we have become impatient, hurried and irritable. Consider this quote from the *Wall Street Journal:* "While impolite behavior has always been a fact of life, there is mounting evidence that incivility not only is on the rise but has become almost the norm in many parts of our culture. A recent University of North Carolina survey of 775 workers nationwide found that every single person had experienced some type of rude behavior on the job, including insults, nasty e-mails and denigrating gossip."

You see, all of this contact with people can be quite overwhelming. Stimulating. Even nerve-racking.

Our nervous systems were created in a simpler time. The world of our ancestors, the world that existed for

7 million years, as our nervous system was formed, was free of electronic gadgets. It was free of motors and motorized noises. And it was free of voices and images communicated electronically throughout the day. For the most part, it was a world that was free of the type of stimulating and superficial contact that fills our days.

The world of our ancestors was limited to few people, few human contacts. It has been estimated that our ancestors lived in contact with 150 to 175 people. Most of the people in this group were well known to each other; relatives and members of the same tribe.

The skills, the mind-set, the patterns of relating within this prehistoric society evolved in harmony with the circumstances of life. In balance. While the prehistoric lives of our ancestors were brutish, a subsistence life spent avoiding disease, avoiding hunger, avoiding violent death, it was a predictable life. There were only a small number of people to know. The challenges in life were clearly defined and predictable, following the cycle of the seasons and the changes of weather. It was a balanced and simple life.

Of course you would not want to live this type of life; almost no one would. The thrust of human development has been to creatively escape the brutish, subsistence lives of our ancestors. And we have.

But our brains, our nervous systems, our innate social needs were formed in those times. Strangers were dangerous until proven otherwise. Novelty, unknown sights and sounds, were a threat to the fragile stability of life. In fact, the human nervous system evolved an elaborate and

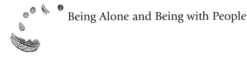

deeply seated alarm system to warn us about dangerous changes in our circumstances.

Social relations were based on mutually shared needs for survival. There was a common foundation of interest, of skills, of communication patterns, of support. Over millions of years, these needs and the interpersonal structures that allowed our ancestors to survive became hardwired into our brains. The patterns of social relatedness that we are born with are the same as those of our prehistoric ancestors. For relationships with people, your brain works with a balance that was developed over millions of years.

- Part of your brain developed to understand social skills, how to relate in the context of your needs, in the context of your life. This is a higher brain function. It balances the stimulation that comes from the following two lower brain centers.
- Part of your brain, a lower brain center, developed to give you a sense of satisfaction and reward when you are relating in the way that works for you. This part of your brain stimulates you to make contact.
- Another part of your brain, located deep within the brain stem, developed to warn you, to alert you to danger, to keep you away from people and circumstances that might harm you. This part of your brain stimulates you to be on guard and perhaps to run away or to fight.

These three parts of your brain operate in a natural balance. From the way that these parts of your brain and mind operate, you can find a pathway to balance. The natural rules of balance that guide your contact with people are natural rules that were formed millions of years ago.

To be in balance, you must recognize the lessons of the past and how they apply to contact with people in our modern life. You can be in balance when you know the rules—how to make contact in a healthy and balanced way.

Read Charlotte's story about the natural rules that she followed to achieve a balance of being with people and being alone.

Feeling Lonely in a Crowd

As a fifth-grade teacher, Charlotte's life was filled with people. Despite this, the reason that she gave for seeking my help was that she was lonely. She worried that she would never be able to find the right man and settle down. Long brown hair, blue eyes, a ready and pleasant smile, her figure was trim from hiking. As though she had absorbed the energy of her students, her personality sparkled with an intelligent curiosity. When I met Charlotte, there was no doubt in my mind that some man would indeed be fortunate to attract her. Still, she had severe doubts about herself. And worry.

"I worry that I'm fat," she told me, when I asked her what was troubling her. "I just don't think I'm pretty enough. I'll never find a man." This was a startling admission from Charlotte. She was, in fact, a beautiful woman. Although Charlotte was a worrier by nature, it seemed to me that her

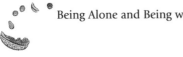

worries about her appearance were unrealistic, perhaps cover-ing some other trouble. We talked about her family.

Charlotte was the youngest of four children. The only girl, Charlotte fit right in with the boys, playing whiffle ball in the backyard, climbing trees, even wrestling with her brothers. Her brothers teased her about how skinny she was, as she tried to keep up and couldn't. From that experience, she resolved to prove her-self; she would show them that she could do anything they did, that she could keep up. Later, when she reached puberty, she and her brothers would spend weekends away from the tensions at home, backpacking and camping in a nearby state forest.

Her dad, a hard-working man, was an auto mechanic. A heavy drinker, he was prone to fits of anger and violence toward the boys, when, after a demanding day, he drank too much. The boys protected Charlotte. At times, there were fights.

As the only female child, Charlotte became a confidant for her mother. Saddened and distraught by the breakdown in her mar-riage, Charlotte's mother would tell her about the misery of mar-riage; about the untrustworthiness of men. "Be your own woman," her mom would tell her. "Don't sacrifice yourself to any man."

Charlotte became a workaholic. It is easy to do when your work is teaching children. She spent long hours preparing for class, long hours providing extra help to the kids who needed it, long hours leading extracurricular activities.

What little time off she had was spent in energetic socializing. Restaurants, movies, the theater with an endless succession of different men. It was exciting, even fun, but she never let any-one get close to her. Her worries would interfere. Did this new man have a drinking problem? Would he be faithful? Would he be successful? Could he possibly be interested in her?

When she was alone, Charlotte watched movies and dreamed. She spent time on the Internet, in chat rooms discussing men. Or when she felt guilty, she would labor over teaching plans for her class.

Even though she was surrounded by people—all day long she was with her students and the other teachers; she dated different men three or four nights per week—Charlotte was convinced that there was something wrong with her. She was lonely, confused and worried.

"I don't know why I feel so lonely," she told me, "I'm with people all of the time." That led to our first rule of balance for Charlotte. Although she had hundreds of contacts per day, she did not have deeper relationships with anyone. We set out to correct this balance problem by creating some rules to guide her.

Charlotte's Rule for Being with People

1. Try to develop deeper relationships with five people. Do this by limiting her superficial social contacts.

Charlotte started with her mother. She sought her out, slowly working to repair the relationship that was destroyed by her father's drinking.

A group of female teachers at school met weekly over lunch. Charlotte asked to join. To her surprise, she found that simply hearing these older women share stories from their lives helped her gain a better sense of how men and women relate.

She cut down on dating. Instead, she spent time with

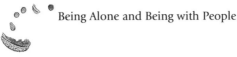
her new friends from the teachers group at school.

Charlotte replaced her chat-room sessions with phone calls to her brothers. From them, she learned more about how they related to their wives and to their families. Her brothers helped her understand how men and women work together in a committed relationship.

Her confidence grew. Through the perspective she gained, Charlotte began to see that, for her, the dating scene was tedious; it left her feeling superficial and somewhat forced. The drinking in the clubs scared her; she felt on guard much of the time. As we talked, Charlotte realized that it was up to her to define what she wanted in a relationship. Based on her past, we came up with some rules.

Charlotte's Rules for Dating

1. *Spend time with men in enjoyable activities like hiking.*
2. *Avoid any man who drinks.*
3. *Look for a man who values her independent style and her professionalism.*
4. *Understand the impact of her appearance on men.*

As she put these rules into practice, Charlotte found that she had more time. Fewer hours were spent dating; more time was spent alone. The dating became more satisfying, although less frequent. But Charlotte found that she prized her time alone. On walks through her neighborhood, Charlotte had the time and space to sort her thoughts out, to make sense of her dating experience, to make up her mind. This became Charlotte's last rule of balance.

Charlotte's Rule for Being Alone

1. *Spend at least two hours per week alone, to relax and to reflect on her experience with men.*

That is how Charlotte established balance. By decreasing overstimulating, unsatisfying contact with people; by replacing it with fewer, deeper and more genuine relationships; by finding time to be alone with her thoughts, to reflect on her experience. In balance, she was able to change her life.

What Is the Balance of Being Alone and Being with People?

People are important. So important that over the millions of years of human development, the human brain has become deeply involved with social functioning. There is no other human function that is so deeply wired into the brain. There is no other human function that occupies so much of the brain. Nothing else that we think or do is as important as social function.

Medical researchers are now discovering that human relatedness and social function are two of the most important factors in promoting health and well-being. The health benefits of close relationships with people include: preventing depression, improving recovery from cancer, decreasing heart disease and stroke, lowering blood pressure. When you have close and healthy relationships with people your immune system is better at fighting infection; you become more resilient; your productivity for school and work increases. Your brain, your body and your mind all function better with the right amount of healthy relationships with people.

How much contact is healthy? What type of contact? What characterizes a relationship that is health-promoting? It is now possible to be clear about the facts. Some hard-nosed science can guide us.

Here are the facts:

- Our brains developed over the ages to handle only about 200 to 250 relationships of all types. More than this, and your nervous system can be overloaded. Since all of us are exposed to more people than this through direct contact, through the media and through electronic forms of communication, a certain amount of overstimulation is a part of our culture.
- Close relationships promote health and well-being. Researchers have found people who have five or more close relationships experience significant health benefits.
- Close relationships that promote health have the following characteristics: empathy and mutual understanding; acceptance; warmth; emotional support; a sense that you can confide in each other; and trust.

- Negative relationships are harmful to your brain. Being exposed to anger, violence, excessive criticism and danger leads to lasting changes in your brain that make you more vulnerable to depression and anxiety.
- Your brain is innately wired to recognize healthy relationships and unhealthy relationships. When you are in healthy contact with people, neural pathways are activated that are health-promoting, that provide you with a sense of satisfaction and reward. When you are in an unhealthy relationship, your brain becomes alarmed and you become nervous, stressed, even depressed.
- You learn good social skills; you learn good people skills through experience and through the positive impact of other people. It takes work and thought to figure it out. Being good with people doesn't just happen: You have to think about it; you have to learn it.

The fact is that we are spending too much time in a kind of unhealthy alone state. When you watch television or movies you are alone. When you sit at your computer, sending e-mail or surfing the Internet, you are alone. When you sit on the crowded subway or on a bus you are alone. Unless you bring a friend, when you shop in the malls, you are alone. Many of the modern inventions that have enriched our lives have also caused a fundamental change in how we relate to people. More and more of our time is spent in contact with people we don't really know; our days are filled to excess with superficial contacts,

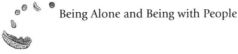

vibrant images of attractive people, with media portrayals of people in overly dramatic situations. And as we live through this flood of contact each day, we are alone.

The new technologies shift the way that we relate, sacrificing deeper ties and meaningful contact and replacing them with rapid and abundant connections. At the same time, the social context of human contact is lost. We have replaced warmth, empathy and mutual support with speed, sound bytes, drama and excitement. It is almost impossible to connect in a deep way by e-mail. It is just too quick. Watching endless television provides the images and the drama of human life without the reassurance that can only come from a deeper relationship. Spending too much time alone, surfing the Internet, can make you depressed and anxious.

Your brain works in a balance. The stimulation of new people and changing events is balanced by the calming reassurance of close human contact. It is balanced by time spent alone, in reflection. Being exposed to endless, impersonal and novel human contact—as we all are in modern life—puts us in a situation of imbalance. Our brains become stimulated by the contact; the lower centers of our brains are stimulated selectively; we end up feeling excited and entertained, or worried and unsettled. Lacking a deeper connection, in the absence of human social context, you do not have the natural tools to quiet this excitement—without the right balance of deeper ties and time spent in reflection, we live, over time, with only the unsettling effects of life spent in the moment.

This can leave you feeling overwhelmed, stressed,

overstimulated. It can seem as though there are too many people in your life and that you need to get away. In reality, we are alone too much. Modern life has, little by little, pushed close and meaningful human contact from our day-to-day lives. We are not able to spend enough time with our circle of friends and family, that group of people with whom we have supportive and mutually sustaining relationships. Instead, we are surrounded by a sea of people we don't know. We are alone with a flood of strangers—every day.

A real paradox of modern life is that while we spend so much of our time alone with a stimulating barrage of superficial human contact, many of us do not have time for a healthy type of being alone. What is healthy aloneness? It is time spent by yourself, away from the modern stimulation of television, movies, city crowds and computers. All of these modern situations tap right into your awareness and prevent you from being alone with your thoughts.

Instead, you are alone with external stimulation. To be truly alone, in a healthy way, you must spend time relaxed, not tensely awaiting the next intrusion into your personal space. To be alone in a healthy way, you must have the time and space to think and to reflect. For this is the way that you learn, especially about people. You must have a chance to be alone with your thoughts; to sort out your reactions and to reflect on a course of action.

One byproduct of modern life is the loss of balance. We spend so much time in contact with others, communicating, commuting, watching and shopping, that we don't have time for the essential human activities

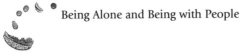

of connecting deeply with people we care about and spending time alone in thoughtful reflection.

How to Balance Time with People and Time Alone

Here are four natural rules to follow, based on the way that your brain works in balance. Use these rules to help balance the amount of time you spend with people and the amount of time you spend alone.

Rule #1: Find a Way to Spend Time Alone

This means without the telephone the television, your computer or your cell phone. As a rule of thumb, you will need about two hours per week to think about people. Spend this time reviewing your experiences with the people you care about. Think about ways to relate that are more satisfying and helpful. Strategize about what you may need to do, to be better with people and to feel better treated. Be sure to think positively and to limit the time. Too much time spent reflecting, especially when that time is spent in self-criticism, is not helpful. It may be useful to spend your alone time engaging in an activity that reduces tension. This will help you think more clearly.

Rule #2: Work Actively to Maintain at Least Five Close Relationships

This does not have to be a burden. It can be a joy. Find the time for this health-giving activity by cutting back on superficial contacts. Your close relationships should be characterized by empathy, trust, warmth, acceptance, emotional support and a feeling that you can confide in each other.

Rule #3: Foster Relationships That Feel Right; End the Ones That Don't

Your brain is wired in such a way that a healthy relationship feels right; it will feel rewarding, satisfying and calming. On the other hand, an unhealthy relationship does not feel right; it can feel hurtful, stressful and demanding. As you spend time reflecting, check your gut reactions. Ask yourself if you feel good about a particular relationship or not. When you do this, you are using tools that nature has given you to size up your situation. Your brain is doing it anyway, so you might as well get the benefit of tuning in to your brain's instinctive responses. Then, work on keeping the healthy relationships and ending the relationships that are not.

Rule #4: Spend at Least an Hour Per Day Away from All Forms of Superficial, Stimulating Contact

Use this time to relax and recharge your batteries. Remember, all of the superficial contacts with people are actually charging your nervous system with energy of a sort; your brain interprets the novelty, the change and the lack of human warmth as a danger signal. It can be stressful. So, for an hour per day, shut off your cell phone, turn

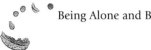

off the TV, log off the Internet; spend some time either alone or in the company of someone you love. Sleep, write, exercise, sing or walk; any activity will do as long as it is free of superficial, stimulating contact. You may want to use this time to add some healthy movement to your life. This will have the added benefit of helping you think.

How Should You Spend Your Time with People?

A woman I know loves horses. Any activity related to horses and horseback riding is a pleasure for my friend Vanessa. She loves the joyful beauty of riding a horse. The experience of caring for, working with and being around horses connects to who she is quite unlike anything else in her life. Naturally enough, Vanessa has formed deep and enduring relationships with people as a result of her love for horses. She and her husband met at a riding event. Vanessa's dear friends all share her love of horses. Her children ride with her and help care for the horses they all love. Every close relationship in Vanessa's life contains this common thread.

My life has been enriched through a deep connection to athletics. It might be ice hockey or skiing or hiking; as long as the activity involves the rhythmic pleasures of athletic exertion I'm happy. And so I have formed many deep and lasting relationships through athletics. My wife and I first fell in love as we hiked through the White Mountains together. When my partner and I talk, we do so during a game of squash or on the golf course. I cherish the time I spend with my father on the golf course. It works for me. It feels right.

What works for you? What is the natural path to follow, the natural flowing way for you to be with people and to form lasting relationships? How do you make sense of the world and the people in it? Since close relationships are essential to balance, asking these questions can lead you to a healthy balance.

What's more, these questions are important because of the way that your brain works. There is no one right way to form a close and healthy relationship but there is a way for you to do so that is uniquely suited to who you are. When you follow your own natural rhythms, then relationships form quickly. They last longer. They can be more satisfying and rewarding to you. Spending time with people in a manner that fits who we are is a natural antidote to our hurried, impersonal and disconnected modern lives.

Here is how it works. The thinking part of your brain, the higher centers of your mind, located in the right frontal lobes, help you relate to people. This part of your brain reads the language of interactions with people and tells you what is happening. To do this, the right part of your brain uses the tools at hand, the neural pathways that you were born with. Everyone is different. Everyone processes information in a slightly different way. So the right part of your brain uses the information-processing pathways that are unique to you, to read other people; to interpret social interactions, to relate in a comfortable manner. The styles of information processing can be grouped into several categories.

Educators have understood this for many years, speaking in terms of different types of intelligence as a foundation for learning. Nowadays, educators attempt to tailor the curricula in schools to the unique *intelligence* for each child, to the unique style of learning.

Of course, you have a unique style of information processing! Some people are musical, some people are oriented toward reading and words, some people understand the world through movement. Ponder on this for a minute, and you can see that it is common sense.

How Your Brain Processes Information

Verbal

Dramatic/Emotional

Visual/Mechanical

Intellectual/Professional

Athletic

Musical

The idea of balance takes this one step further. Like my friend Vanessa, finding a path to balance in relationships works best when you use your natural style of information processing—when you allow your right brain to know about people, to read the grammar of interpersonal relationships, to become close to people by using the information-processing tools that are natural to you, relating to others in a style that feels natural, balanced and comfortable for you.

In the past, for our ancestors, this was an automatic process. For any small group of people, for any village or tribe of one hundred to two hundred people, everyone was a specialist. Everyone could stand out in his or her own way. The best hunter (someone who understood the world through movement) would quickly stand out. The most verbal became the keeper of records, the scribe, the source of community history. Those with intellectual minds became shamans, wise men and village leaders. The village, as a whole, related to each person through the framework of their skills, and each person related to the village through the language of their natural skills.

It is not this way today. With each technological advance, we have become homogenized. As we become part of an ever-larger community, we lose our uniqueness. The world begins to relate to each person as a number, indistinguishable from our neighbors. In the vast sea of humanity, we become no more than our identifying numbers: zip code, Social Security number, income level, education level, telephone number, socioeconomic class. Even our race, our very genetic inheritance is numbered and coded.

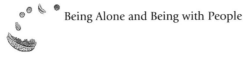

It happens because there are so many of us. It happens because our wonderful inventions were created to provide each of us with abundance. Everyone has the gift of electricity; everyone has access to rich and varied markets; everyone has unlimited access to information.

The unexpected price that we pay is balance. With the homogenization and mass-marketization of our world, we have lost touch with the inborn need to relate to our fellow man in a unique and personal manner. The expectation is that we are all the same. We all watch the news; we all take the same subjects in school, we work in much the same way. In our mass market world, the expectation is that we all relate in the same way—women in book groups, men on the golf course. Everyone is expected to be verbally adept, quick-witted and conversationally fluent. Just like the people on TV. But the biologic fact is that we are not.

Each of us has unique skills and abilities and that is how we can relate in balance. Trying to relate in a mass market way, in sound bytes and witticisms, in a predominantly verbal manner is just not right for everyone. In fact, it is not right for most of us. To develop deeper relationships—the type of relationships that are healthy and which produce balance in life—relate to others in the way that you are made. Use your natural skills to develop close relationships. It works better. It feels better. It leads to balance.

You can do this by following these two rules of balance.

Rule #1: Find Your Natural Style for Processing Information

Verbal

If you are naturally a verbal person, you prefer to relate by talking. Verbal people like to sit and talk. Long dinners, book clubs and one-on-one conversation work well. Verbal people are more likely to enjoy "working the crowd" at parties. The telephone can be a favorite gadget. When it is time to learn something new, verbal people do best when they are "talked through it."

Dramatic/Emotional

If you process information emotionally, you prefer feeling to talking. For you, it's not what people say, it is how they say it. You tune in to the body language, the tone of voice, the emotion of the speaker. Preferred activities are usually intense, with high energy and drama. For example, an emotional person may enjoy whitewater rafting with a group of friends. Or the highs and lows of community theater. Sharing a powerful experience is a way for you to really get to know someone and to feel comfortable with them.

Visual/Mechanical

If you process information visually, you relate by doing. It could be photography, painting or working on a car; what matters is that you can share an experience with someone that involves an activity that you can understand by touching, seeing and manipulating. If this is your style, you will feel most comfortable when you are engaged in a project with someone. Engineers, auto mechanics and visual artists, like photographers and painters, to name a few, tend to be visual/mechanical information processors.

Intellectual/Professional

The world of ideas and analysis tends to characterize those with this style of information processing. It really has nothing to do with IQ. Instead, if this is your style, you become engaged with ideas and analysis; looking at things from all angles. If this is who you are, you may find "small talk" tedious. You prefer to get to the important issues, to discuss things in depth. You will naturally be drawn to academic institutions, and issue-oriented groups where you can engage with others in deep discussion and analysis.

Athletic

Although the common conception of athletes is that they are "dumb jocks," there is a deep and native intelligence, a style of information processing possessed by athletes. Since we humans were created as a hunting species, this may be the most natural, the most deeply wired type of intelligence. If this is your style, you understand life through movement. You relate through movement. And you will form deep relationships through movement, such as sports or dance. If this is who you are, you will find static, slow-moving social engagements to be tiresome and tedious. You will prefer to relate with someone as you move. For that reason, team activities, movement classes such as martial arts, or aerobics or dance may work well for you.

Musical

Of all the informational processing styles, musical information processing is the most commonly understood and accepted as a unique form of interpersonal relating. For that reason, music and social relatedness have a long, well-accepted and widespread history. If you are musical by nature, then you will know what to do. Relate through your music. There are a myriad of opportunities to do so.

This lengthy discussion leads to the next natural rule for guiding how you are with people. By now you will have a pretty good idea of what it is.

Rule #2: Use Your Natural Style of Information Processing to Form Close Relationships

Once you have figured out how you best relate, then you can find a way to do so. That will lead to balance. Relating to others in your natural style will help you form the kind of close relationships that are healthy, the type of close relationships that balance the stimulated, uncomfortable aloneness of modern life. When you follow your natural style you will find that being with people is more comfortable, more satisfying, closer and more in balance.

Here is a story about Robert, and how he followed these two natural rules to establish balance in his life.

"Maybe I'm Not Marriage Material"

The fact that he had never married was a puzzle to Robert. Upsetting, too; he was raised in a large family, and he had many fond memories of life with his brother and sisters. His dream was to marry and raise a family, like the one he had growing up. But as much as he wanted this, it just had not happened for him.

Forty years old and a successful insurance agent, Robert loved selling. He experienced real pleasure from the excitement of meeting new customers and persuading them to buy the right amount of insurance. It was fun for him. It felt good.

When Robert came to see me, his girlfriend Penny had given him an ultimatum. Either marry within the year, or the relationship was over. They had been together for five years. For some reason, the relationship had never progressed beyond their usual pattern of seeing each other on weekends, and on one or two nights during the week.

I asked Robert how he and Penny spent their time.

"Penny loves to eat out in restaurants. When we get together, that's what we do. Or, we spend time at home, playing board games and talking. I love numbers and gambling so I get into playing backgammon together. It helps to pass the time as we talk. After a while, it wears thin, so I usually leave and go home to do some work."

"You don't stay over?" I asked.

"No. Penny feels there are some issues that we have to talk out before we do. I've avoided doing that. I feel guilty about it, but I just can't stomach the idea of sitting down and talking about one issue after another," Robert told me. "I'd rather make some sales calls or do some paperwork. I know that

sounds bad. Maybe I'm just not cut out to be married."

We talked about what Robert liked. What came to him naturally. A risk taker by nature, Robert loved the excitement of
gambling. Smart about money, with a good sense of
perspective, Robert kept his gambling in check. He had always
been able to use it as a source of entertainment, setting aside a
small amount of money to gamble—entertainment money—
Robert would go to a casino for an evening and stay until he
lost his small stake, thoroughly enjoying himself. Penny refused
to go to the casino with him. She felt that gambling was just
not fun, and possibly dangerous. On weekends, Robert loved
new and exciting activities. He had tried parachuting, bungee
jumping and hang-gliding.

Community theater was another passion. Robert was a committed, if somewhat amateur actor. In fact, he had met Penny
at a post-production party, after a successful production of
Fiddler on the Roof.

"Maybe Penny and I don't like the same things," Robert said
sadly, after thinking this through. In fact, in his heart Robert
believed that relationships would always be dull and uninteresting.

*"You know, I kind of dread my time with Penny. That's how
it's always been for me. I do what I think I'm supposed to do,
you know like you see on TV—restaurants, movies, long walks
on the beach to talk—but I end up feeling bored and restless. I
guess I'm hopeless."*

Since he did not really understand himself, Robert had been
unable to develop a close relationship with Penny, or with any
woman. Acting on ideas about how he was supposed to behave
with women, he related in a way that did not fit who he was.
In talking with Robert, it was clear that he preferred a

dramatic/emotional style of interaction, one that was filled with excitement. He mistakenly had tried to relate to Penny, and to most women, in a style that was not suited to him. This led us to formulate rules to guide him.

Robert's Rules for Building Close Relationships

1. *Find his natural style for processing information. By talking about the activities he naturally enjoyed, through a process of self-reflection, Robert discovered that he loved drama, excitement and high risk. This led us to the conclusion that Robert's style of information processing was dramatic/emotional.*

2. *Use his natural style of information processing to develop relationships: Robert thought about his preferences; how he felt most comfortable and natural. This led to some rules to guide him in relationships.*

   - *Build a relationship with someone who has a love for theater.*
   - *Spend time together in exciting activities, like gambling or hang-gliding.*
   - *Find someone who works in sales.*
   - *Don't worry about talking through issues. Do what feels right.*

Having met at a community theater party, Robert assumed that he and Penny had similar interests. But when they talked about it, he discovered that Penny loved the social interactions and the small talk at parties. On the other hand, Robert loved to have a party with people he had just shared an exciting activity with. He and Penny were operating on different scripts.

Breaking a relationship is sad, but as he and Penny became clear about their preferences, they knew it would not work. Although there were many things that they valued about each other, when they were together, Robert and Penny felt out of synch.

They ended the relationship, and after a while they each felt better. Robert fell in love with Ashley, a woman who played lead, opposite him, in a community theater production. He sent me a postcard, from Hawaii. He and Ashley had married, in a ceremony held on a cliff, overlooking the ocean; it was the most famous hang-gliding cliff in Hawaii!

By letting himself follow his natural style, Robert had been able to achieve balance—a healthy relationship with a woman he loved.

Being with People and Being Alone Self-Test

Take this test to see if you are out of balance. If you answer yes to two or more questions, then you may have balance problems with this system. To improve your balance, try to implement the rules in this chapter as well as the tips to follow.

1. In general, do you feel that you are not able to spend enough meaningful and satisfying time with people you care about each day?   yes   no
2. Do you spend more time communicating with others by phone, voice mail or computer than you do in person?   yes   no
3. Each day, do you spend more time watching people on television, in movies and on the computer than you do relating to people you care about?   yes   no
4. Do you feel that you have no one to turn to for advice and guidance?   yes   no

Tips to Balance Being with People and Being Alone

Try incorporating some of these tips in your life over the next week to help yourself begin to find a healthy balance of being with people and being alone. Or use the tips to trigger your thoughts, and then create some tips that work uniquely for you.

1. Take a hot bath and use the time in the tub to think about the people you care about. Don't answer the phone, turn off the radio, don't watch TV. Let the gentle warmth of the water help you to relax as you take a few moments to be alone with your thoughts.

2. Handwrite brief notes to your friends instead of using the telephone or e-mail. Taking the time to write your thoughts and wishes will strengthen the bond of friendship. The act of writing helps you to think while also reducing your stress levels.

3. Tell someone you like why you like them. Tell your friend or loved one why they are important to you and what you value in the relationship. This can feel quite nice. Explaining why you like someone also helps you by creating a positive memory or a positive image of that person.

4. Fill out the worksheet starting on page 77, to better understand your natural style of information processing.

5. Take one activity from the information processing worksheet, the activity with the most "enjoyable" checkmarks, and make a plan to do that activity with someone you like.

6. Share a relaxed meal with a friend or with your family. Try to do this at least once a week.

7. Find a group of people who like what you like and meet with them on a regular basis. It could be a sewing group, a book group, an exercise class, a political committee or a fantasy football league. What matters is that you meet regularly with people who have the same interests as you.

8. Go for a drive, by yourself, on a quiet scenic road. When you do, shut off your cell phone, shut off your pager, keep the radio turned off. Use the time in your car to relax and think about the people in your life.

If you commute to and from work, pick a special, relaxing route home from work. Then use your drive home to reflect on the people in your day.

9. Learn to say no in a nice way. When you are asked to do something that feels like an imposition; when you feel someone does not have your best interests in mind; when being with a particular person leaves you feeling unsettled; figure out how to say no. Just like everything in life, some relationships are healthy and some are not. It's not anyone's fault, but if a relationship is unhealthy, then it is best to say no.

10. Give your relationship a voice—a creative way to express your affection. You can do this a number of ways. Read out loud to your children, your family or your friends. Sing or play music. Dance. Work on a project together. Go to church services together. Move and be athletic together. Cook together. Create a garden with someone you love. Any activity that allows you to express yourself can be a vehicle for strengthening a relationship.

INFORMATION PROCESSING WORKSHEET

Check the box that best describes your feeling about each activity. Incorporate the activities you find most enjoyable into your life.

	NEVER ENJOYABLE	RARELY ENJOYABLE	SOMETIMES ENJOYABLE	OFTEN ENJOYABLE	USUALLY ENJOYABLE	ALWAYS ENJOYABLE
VERBAL						
Cocktail parties						
Talking on the phone						
Talking with your spouse						
Writing letters						
Social clubs						
Dining with friends						
Small talk						
Working meetings						
Local politics						
Book group						

INFORMATION PROCESSING WORKSHEET *(continued)*

	NEVER ENJOYABLE	RARELY ENJOYABLE	SOMETIMES ENJOYABLE	OFTEN ENJOYABLE	USUALLY ENJOYABLE	ALWAYS ENJOYABLE
DRAMATIC/EMOTIONAL						
Intense relationships						
High-risk activities						
Acting or performing in public						
Powerful feelings						
Gambling						
Shopping						
Surprise parties						
Soap operas						
Sharing "peak" experiences						
Reading romance/ mystery novels						

INFORMATION PROCESSING WORKSHEET (*continued*)

	NEVER ENJOYABLE	RARELY ENJOYABLE	SOMETIMES ENJOYABLE	OFTEN ENJOYABLE	USUALLY ENJOYABLE	ALWAYS ENJOYABLE
VISUAL/MECHANICAL						
Hobbies or crafts						
Painting or photography						
Working on cars						
Home projects						
Going to art museums						
Decorating your home						
Craft clubs						
Woodworking						
Sewing, quilting or knitting						
Gardening						

INFORMATION PROCESSING WORKSHEET *(continued)*

	NEVER ENJOYABLE	RARELY ENJOYABLE	SOMETIMES ENJOYABLE	OFTEN ENJOYABLE	USUALLY ENJOYABLE	ALWAYS ENJOYABLE
INTELLECTUAL/PROFESSIONAL						
Learning and academics						
Educational meetings						
TV news and history shows						
Debating issues						
Reading nonfiction						
Attending lectures						
Cause-oriented groups						
Browsing in book shops						
Discussing ideas						
Researching ideas						

INFORMATION PROCESSING WORKSHEET *(continued)*

ATHLETIC	NEVER ENJOYABLE	RARELY ENJOYABLE	SOMETIMES ENJOYABLE	OFTEN ENJOYABLE	USUALLY ENJOYABLE	ALWAYS ENJOYABLE
Dance, figure skating or gymnastics						
Sports (tennis, golf, softball)						
Martial arts						
Aerobics						
Team athletics						
Talking while walking						
Working out						
Staying in shape						
Watching sports						
Watching dance or ballet						

INFORMATION PROCESSING WORKSHEET *(continued)*

	NEVER ENJOYABLE	RARELY ENJOYABLE	SOMETIMES ENJOYABLE	OFTEN ENJOYABLE	USUALLY ENJOYABLE	ALWAYS ENJOYABLE
MUSICAL						
Playing music						
Listening to music						
Music lessons						
Musical theater						
Singing						
Symphony						
Opera						
Choral groups						
Playing in a band						
Composing music						

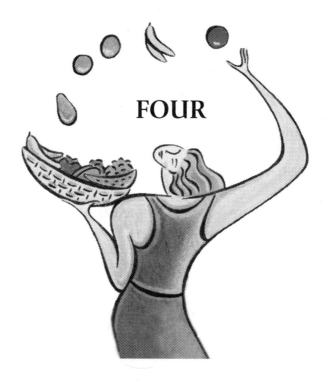

FOUR

System 2:
Movement and Rest

Since World War II, we have been busy engineering physical activity out of daily life.

Steven N. Blair, research director at the Cooper Institute,
quoted in the *Wall Street Journal*, May 1, 2000

We human beings are a mobile, restless, active species. We were created to be in motion, not to rest. Live with a natural and healthy balance of movement and rest and your life will have a melody to it; your life will have a balanced phrasing; your life will move in harmonious rhythms.

Movement helps your brain to think.

By linking the energy and emotion of the lower centers of your brain with thought from the higher centers of your mind, movement produces a flowing and rhythmic process of thinking and feeling. Healthy movement is a natural antidote for the immobile but overstimulated style of life today. It helps your brain and mind translate the instinctive energy of your older brain—energy that is sparked by the excitement and stimulation of our modern technologies. Movement turns instinctive energy into flowing thought.

But if you do not move enough, if you lose the balance of movement and rest, the music stops. When you lose the balance of movement and rest you lose the music of life; that fluid, dynamic harmonious processing; the *flow* that you feel when you are happy and healthy. When you do not have the right balance of movement and rest, here is what can happen to you:

- a block in your thinking (like writer's block),
- a sense that life is overwhelming,
- a feeling that you cannot solve your problems,
- a tendency toward being overly self-conscious,
- a feeling that you are not comfortable in your own skin,

- a feeling of restless uneasiness,
- overly sensitive and reactive to people,
- tiredness and lassitude that results in trouble getting motivated,
- muscle stiffness, cramping and achiness,
- joint stiffness and pain, poor sleep.

Do you have enough movement in your life? Or is your life overbalanced toward inactivity? Answer the following questions to find out.

1. Do you get less than thirty minutes of physical activity per day?	yes	no
2. Do exercise vigorously less than three times per week?	yes	no
3. Do you prefer to drive everywhere you go while avoiding walking?	yes	no
4. Do you have trouble getting yourself off of the couch?	yes	no
5. Do you avoid physical activity because you feel tired all of the time?	yes	no
6. Have you given up on trying to exercise?	yes	no
7. Do you become tired or get short of breath after a brief period of physical activity?	yes	no
8. Do you feel restless, edgy or uptight at the end of the day?	yes	no
9. Do you suffer with tension headaches?	yes	no
10. Do you suffer with muscle tension, muscle aches or pain?	yes	no
11. Do you suffer with lower back pain?	yes	no
12. Are you a restless sleeper?	yes	no
13. Do you have trouble relaxing?	yes	no

If you answered yes to five or more of these questions, you may be out of balance. It could well be that, like all of us, you need more healthy movement in your life. If that is the case, take heart, there is a lot you can do. As you read this chapter, you will learn about some natural rules for living that will guide you to a healthy balance of movement and rest. Put these rules to work and you can feel quite a bit better.

Listen to Ellen's story. In her words, you can hear the way in which modern life can upset your balance. In her story, you can hear the way that she fixed this problem by reestablishing a healthy balance of movement and rest in her life.

Her Only Exercise
Is Chauffeuring the Kids

"I was fine when the kids were younger," Ellen told me. "When they were toddlers I was on my feet all day, pushing them in a stroller, chasing after them, going to the park. You know what it's like. With little ones, you never stop moving. And I had three in five years. You know, it was fun. And tiring. I slept like a log in those days.

"Now my three are all teenagers, thirteen, fourteen and sixteen. The things they are into! My sixteen-year-old is on a traveling baseball team. The girls are into dance, gymnastics and sleepovers. Any time they want to see their friends, I have to drive them. It seems like I'm in the car from seven in the morning until ten at night.

"At home, the two girls want to sit and talk to me. I help them with their homework. I help them figure out how to deal

*with their friends and with boys. By the end of the evening,
I'm exhausted. I collapse in front of the television and watch
whatever is on. Or I call my sister on the West Coast, just to
chat. The only time I get out is for my book group. You know,
we sit around, pretend to talk about a book, but really we talk
about our families."*

*She continued, "Then about three years ago, I started to
have these problems. I'm not the angry type, but still, I was
more impatient with my friends and with Tom. Then my sleep
changed. I'd wake up all the time. Three or four times a night.
I never felt rested. All I wanted to do was to lie down. Last year,
I thought I had arthritis. My joints hurt all the time. I went to
the doctor, but he said there was nothing wrong. But if there is
nothing wrong, why do I feel so crummy?"*

Ellen is a good mom. She loves her kids. She will do
anything for them. It is heartwarming to talk with her, to
experience the way that she has given herself, heart and
soul, to her children.

That is how she lost her balance. Through her devotion
to her children, she stopped providing for herself. It is a
problem that many parents share.

We talked about the times in her life that she felt healthy,
the times when she felt well. Ellen had been a dancer when
she was a girl. As a teenager, she danced at least four nights
per week. There were lessons, recitals and just dancing for
pleasure. Ellen recalled the rhythmic motion, in a flow with
the music. While dancing, she felt the athletic pleasure of
her muscles at work. Her mind, engaged with the music
and the movement, felt relaxed and alive.

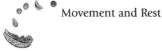

She continued to dance until she married and started to have kids. Then, there was just not enough time. On the rare occasions that she and her husband could get away to dance, she could, for an evening, recapture the joy and peace of movement.

As we talked, it became clear to Ellen that she lost touch with a natural rule of balance in her life: She did not have enough healthy movement in her life.

Ellen and I worked to correct this situation. We figured out how to free up some time. This is always the first step. Then Ellen found a path to movement. Middle-aged, she no longer felt comfortable in a dance class with lithe adolescents. She decided to take a tai chi class given at her church. She also found time to sing in the choir at her church.

Her family had to help. Her kids and her husband pitched in to take care of some household chores. Her kids tried a little harder to make do without homework help. Gradually, she found more time for her tai chi; for her singing. This turned out to be a hidden benefit for Ellen. As her kids and her husband pitched in, she relaxed a bit; she gained confidence in them. She began to feel comfortable with the idea that it was okay to take some time for herself.

The rhythmic stretching of the tai chi worked wonders. For Ellen, it recalled the graceful poses of dance. It made her more flexible; her muscles toned up. The aches and pains began to disappear.

Singing gave her peace of mind. As she joined in the communal harmonies of the church hymns she could feel herself let go of her worries; she could feel her tension melt away. Often as she sang, her mind working in synch with the music, Ellen found new perspective on some of the troubles in her life. As she followed her rule for living, as she reestablished her healthy balance of movement and rest, she found it easier to be a mom.

Movement Is Life

Movement begins shortly after conception. The human fetus is in constant motion within the womb. Movement does not stop until you die. Movement is life.

Every fiber of our being developed according to this guiding principle: Movement is life, prolonged rest is dangerous. If you are too much at rest, alarm bells go off. If you are too much at rest, your body rebels. If you are too much at rest, the beautiful synergy of body and mind is disrupted. If you are too much at rest, as Ellen says, "It feels crummy."

In chapter 2, you learned about the elegant simplicity of your movement center. This simple but elegant balance system was used by nature to control, time and pace all activity within your brain. It is central to the healthy functioning of your brain, your body and your mind. The brain mechanisms that control movement also control the flow of your emotions and the flow of your thoughts.

When you do function with a healthy balance of movement and rest, then your life will flow. As Ellen did, you will find that it becomes easier to think through situations and to solve problems. You will find that it is easier to interact in harmony with other people. You will find it easier to become involved and to stay involved with the parts of life that really matter. You will feel better physically. Healthier. Happier. Contentment and true rest comes more easily when you have the proper balance of movement and rest.

Does this sound remarkable to you? It is. Your brain, mind and body perform as a beautifully synchronized machine when you have the right balance of movement and rest. Nature has provided you with the physical tools to do so. The natural way that this occurs is truly remarkable, a miracle of creation. Understand this, and you will see why I say that movement is life.

How Your Brain Controls Movement: The Music of Your Mind

In the center of your brain is a collection of nerve cells—your movement center. In medical terms, these cells are called the basal ganglia and the cerebellum. Using the balanced process of excitation and inhibition, these cells control the flow of activity in your brain and in your mind; they produce the music of your mind.

The flow of movement, the flow of thought, the flow of language, the flow of emotion, the flow of ideas and the flow of creativity: All are controlled by your movement center. There are neurological connections from your movement centers to all parts of your brain that allow this to happen.

The process begins with a status report from your body. Sensation from every part of your body is sent to your movement center, so that your movement center can figure out what is happening to you. Are you walking? Running? Sitting or lying down? Are you loose and relaxed? Are you tense and uptight? Are you hot or cold? Are you full of energy? Are you tired? Are you happy, sad, angry or worried? Your movement center continuously queries your entire body to answer the question—how am I doing and what am I doing?

When someone asks you "How are you?" and you answer fine, or not so well, or tired or happy or whatever, you are giving a report based on the information collected by your movement center.

Your movement center feeds this report up to the higher centers in your brain—located in your neocortex—where a decision is made about what you should do. Your neocortex will decide what activity should take place, such as, should you run, should you be angry, should you come up with some ideas to solve a problem. This decision is then fed back down to your movement center, where the process of your response is controlled. Your movement center takes the command from above and controls the rhythm, the timing and the pace of your response. Your movement center conducts and directs your activity so that there is a music-like rhythm and flow to your actions.

It all happens lightning fast, with elegant timing and with flow. Your movement center controls the flow of your behavior, and it also tells you about how well you are doing. It operates according to the principle that moving, smooth, fluid and rhythmic activity is good and that immobility—halting, interrupted, spasmodic activity—is not right. And when you are immobile for long periods, then it sends out warning signals that something is amiss.

That is the music of your mind. Reflect on it. You can see the beauty of the system. You sense your internal and external environment. You formulate a response. Then your movement center takes over, conducting, directing and processing to make sure that you respond at the right time, with the right force and with the correct pace.

For our ancestors, movement was life. Think about life in those times. If you wanted or needed anything, you had to move. You had to move to get water, to obtain food, to find shelter, to hear the news from other members of your village. If you needed a tool to grind corn, or to use as a weapon, you had to use your hands to make it. And movement meant survival. At times, it was necessary to move to be safe from dangerous animals, to be safe from warring tribes, to be safe from the dangers of the extremes of weather. Over the eons, your brain developed in such a way that effective and efficient movement was interpreted by your brain as a good sign, as a healthy sign, as a sign that things would work out. On the other hand, if you were not moving, your brain learned to interpret this as a sign of trouble. You might have been sick, you might have been in danger and scared stiff, you might have been unable to leave your home because of a terrible storm, or you might have been old and infirm, a burden to your village.

Here is the part that confuses we modern humans. To the workings of your brain, all types of movement provide the music for your mind. *All types of movement.* It is fashionable to say that the problem of modern life is that we do not get enough vigorous exercise. To a certain extent, that is true. But the real problem is that, when it comes to movement, modern life is out of balance. There is not enough movement of all types to balance our long periods of inactivity. Vigorous exercise is an important factor, there is no doubt about this fact. But so is rhythmic movement, like dance. So is skilled hand movement like sewing. Having a proper balance of movement and rest involves using enough different kinds of motion to balance periods of inactivity.

Why? Because movement helps you think better. A natural rule of human life is that movement controls the flow of energy from the lower centers of your brain to the higher centers, where it is turned into flowing and energetic thought. Movement helps you process your emotions better. Movement helps you to feel better, because your brain was created to function best when there is a healthy amount of movement in your life.

When there is a balance of movement and rest, then the magic happens—you live with a musical rhythm, a natural balance, a flow of energy and thought.

What Is the Natural Balance of Movement and Rest?

To understand the balance of movement and rest, it is necessary to break movement down into two large categories: exercise or vigorous physical activity, and rhythmic movement. Exercise or vigorous physical activity is the type of movement that we all think of as a "workout." Any movement or activity that makes your heart beat, your lungs pump and which causes you to break out into a sweat could be described as exercise.

Rhythmic movement is any activity that causes you to move in a rhythm, with timing, with pace and with flow. It could be singing or tai chi, as it was for Ellen; it could be dance; it could be skiing; or it could be working with your lathe, your router, or your sewing machine. It could be writing letters, painting pictures or swimming. So long as there is a music to your movement, then it fits the definition of rhythmic movement.

It will quickly occur to you that certain kinds of rhythmic movement also make your heart pound, your lungs pump. Certain kinds of rhythmic movement, like a good aerobics class, can really make you sweat. So much the better. The two categories are not mutually exclusive. Rather, both categories are essential ingredients to a healthy balance.

Rest, as I define it, is very different from inactivity. Healthful rest is part of movement. Once you have moved enough, once you have gotten your essential quotient of physical exercise; once you have had enough rhythmic

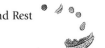

movement to process your thoughts, to process your feelings, to reassure your psyche that everything will be alright, then you rest. Why? You rest as a natural process of restoration, renewal and recovery *so then you can start to move again*. If you have enough movement in your life, then your rest will be relaxing and peaceful.

Now contrast this with inactivity. When you are driving a car, or watching TV, or surfing the Internet, or talking on the phone or riding in a plane, you are not at rest. During these activities, your brain and your mind are subject to an amazing amount of stimulation. You are not at rest during these activities; *you are inactive*. And it is not restful. It can, in fact, make you tense, anxious and wired. All of our life-changing technologies can destroy the balance of movement and rest by replacing movement with an unsettling mix of mental stimulation and physical inactivity.

In order to achieve a healthy, natural balance of movement and rest, it is necessary to have enough physical exercise and rhythmic movement in your life. This leads to the natural rule about exercise.

Rule #1: Get Thirty Minutes of Vigorous Exercise at Least Three Times Per Week

This has been researched over and over by exercise physiologists. If you exercise vigorously this amount or more, the payoff for your health is tremendous. Vigorous exercise is when your heart beats fast, you breathe hard and you sweat. You will lose weight, increase your energy level, lower your blood pressure, improve your mood, sleep better, decrease worry and nervousness and lower your risk of heart disease. You will improve your sense of well-being.

Everyone knows this, but almost no one exercises this much. The U.S. Department of Health and Human Services reports that only 15 percent of Americans get this amount of exercise. And, unless you exercise vigorously for thirty minutes, three times per week, you will be out of balance. Too much inactivity, too little healthful rest.

Why don't more people exercise? The answer lies in the balance of energy and thought; the answer lies in the natural rules of balance that guide the functioning of your mind.

If you approach exercise as a physical chore, then that is what it becomes. But if you use your mind; if the physical act of exercise is linked to thoughts and feelings that matter to you, then your body and your mind operate in harmony.

Let's face facts. If an activity is dull, uninteresting or not meaningful, it can be impossible to do. Consider this question: Why did our ancestors get so much physical exercise? The answer: because they had to, or they would not survive! For our ancestors, physical exercise was essential to life, so of course they exercised. It was a life-or-death matter. And nothing motivates you quite as well as a matter of life and death.

Bring this idea to the present, and you have the underpinnings of some rules for living. To motivate yourself to get enough vigorous exercise, the type of exercise you choose must matter to you in some way. As was true for our ancestors, in order to take on the work of physical exercise, there must be a good reason to do so. Thankfully, these days, your life does not usually depend on the amount of physical exercise you get day to day. So it is necessary to use your mind, to discover other motivating factors. These factors become your rules for living—the rules that will help you establish and maintain a natural balance of movement and rest. The rules will come from answering this question: *What type of activity is interesting, fun or rewarding for me?* That is how you exercise in a balance with your mind. As we saw in the last chapter, there are helpful rules to follow. In just the same way that you follow the rules set by your natural style of information processing, to guide you in forming relationships, you can help yourself get healthy exercise by using a style of exercise that naturally fits who you are. By linking the work of physical exercise with an activity that is fun, interesting or rewarding for you, by getting vigorous physical exercise in a way that is tailored to who you are.

This leads to the next natural rule for balancing movement and rest:

Rule #2: Use Your Natural Style and Preference to Create a Program of Exercise That Is Fun, Interesting or Rewarding

Here are some questions you can use to help you to discover your natural exercise preferences.

1. Do you enjoy, and are you good at, activities that require eye-hand coordination like tennis or softball?   yes   no

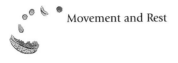
2. Do you enjoy, and are you good at activities that require whole-body movement like skating, gymnastics, dance or horseback riding?   yes   no

3. Do you prefer to exercise with others?   yes   no

4. Do you like to exercise in a class, such as dance, aerobics or martial arts?   yes   no

5. Do you enjoy high-stimulation exercise such as rock climbing, skiing or mountain biking?   yes   no

6. Do you enjoy competing?   yes   no

7. Do you get satisfaction from endurance activities, like running, swimming and triathlons?   yes   no

8. Does music help you exercise?   yes   no

9. Do you prefer to exercise while engaging in an activity that has another purpose, such as gardening or home repair/ construction?   yes   no

---

Any question with a yes answer tells you the way to exercise. A yes answer tells you that a particular form of exercise appeals to you; it is motivating; it engages your mind to work in fluid harmony with your body. You can turn these questions into some effective rules for living. Remember your yes answers and put these rules to work for you, so that you can get enough healthy exercise. Then you can truly rest.

To give you a picture of how this works, read this story about Bob.

His Mind Races, His Body Rests

When Bob came to see me he was miserable. After working too many long hours in his marketing job for a major oil company, he found himself in the middle of a divorce that he really did not understand. Still in love with his wife and devoted to his daughter, Bob couldn't see that he wasn't home enough, that he had become impatient and hard to live with, that he didn't listen to his wife or his daughter. When his wife pressed for a divorce it came as a shock.

Living alone, after the separation, Bob still worked too much. He had never even found the time to unpack the boxes from his move. He was sad and tired all of the time. Bob found it impossible to do anything but work or lay in bed watching movies, while his mind raced.

We talked about some concrete steps he could take to feel better. Exercise was one. But, as you might imagine, the thought of dragging himself out of bed to a gym to push himself to work out seemed overwhelming.

So I changed the subject, and we talked about what Bob could possibly find interesting. We did this to help Bob to follow the rule for living about exercise preferences. He was lonely. He missed his wife and daughter. The single greatest motivator for him was to find a way to spend some time with a friendly female companion. Having played the piano throughout his life, Bob loved music. Listening to music helped him do anything, from balancing his checkbook to painting the house. He liked the idea of endurance activities, of challenging his ability to push himself physically. These factors led him to his exercise preferences.

Bob's exercise preferences:
1. Exercise with people, preferably a woman (at least at this time in his life).
2. Include music.
3. Exercise for endurance.

From these preferences, Bob developed two ideas. Joining a bicycle club, to bicycle long distances, and hiring a personal trainer to help him to get an endurance-type, aerobic workout. A compact CD player and headphones could provide music while he was riding his bike. Since the personal trainer came to his apartment, he could use his stereo system to provide the music for his workout.

Bob started with an early morning workout at home with a personal trainer. This allowed him to fit in the exercise, without cutting back on work. He found the effervescent enthusiasm of his personal trainer so enjoyable, that he actually looked forward to his workouts with pleasure. After a time, his work efficiency improved. He felt more energetic and more clear-headed. He was able to talk reasonably with his ex-wife once again. Although he was still in pain from the divorce, Bob decided he would try to correct some of the shortcomings that had ruptured his marriage.

As he got in shape, as his body responded to the workouts, firming up, gaining energy, Bob found that his confidence increased. Many of the circumstances that had gotten under skin just did not bother him to the same degree. He could face the issues with his wife and daughter without reacting in a negative or self-critical way.

Together he and his ex-wife worked out a way for Bob to spend more time with his daughter. Bob found that his relationship with Hannah took on a new meaning for both of them as Bob introduced Hannah to the activities he enjoyed. He and Hannah joined a bicycle club for fun. Each weekend, they went on bicycle trips with the club. They both thoroughly enjoyed the exercise and the company. Bob took Hannah to concerts. He began to teach her to play the cello, his favorite instrument. Their relationship flourished.

By working out, by getting enough vigorous exercise, Bob reestablished a natural balance in his life. His path to doing this, his natural rules, helped guide him to a type of exercise that he could actually get himself to do. As the weeks passed, as the exercise worked its magic, he gained confidence and he felt better.

Movement Creates Thought

Let's shift into some new territory. Everyone is familiar with the fact that we do not get enough physical exercise, but that is just scratching the surface. The fact is that we are starved for another type of movement—for rhythmic, melodic, musical movement. Movement that has a timing to it, a pace and a flow; movement that has a musical pattern. Movement that follows a flowing script.

Here is a brief list of movement activities that are rhythmic, musical or melodic:

- dance
- skiing
- yoga
- playing a musical instrument
- singing
- painting a picture
- sculpting or pottery making
- writing by hand
- woodworking
- sewing
- rocking in a chair
- juggling
- riding a horse

The list is practically endless. The requirements are simple: The activity must include movement; the movement must be rhythmic in some way, with timing, pace and flow such that the elements of motion are linked together in a pattern or a script that exists in your mind.

There is broad agreement among neuroscientists that your brain learns to think and speak by first learning to move. When the fetus moves in the womb, it creates the brain pathways that will later turn into conscious thought. You may have noticed this same phenomenon in the way that children learn fine hand and finger movements just before they learn to talk. That is the same process at work. There is also strong evidence that our ancestors learned to talk as a result of learning to use tools skillfully. The theory is that the sequence of linked, rhythmic movements of the hand, necessary for tool use, formed the brain pathways that are used by the brain to create language and sophisticated thought. Finally, there is good evidence that movement, specifically movement that occurs when you feel an emotion, is used by the brain to understand and interpret emotional reactions.

The way that this all occurs is that the music of the movement, the timing, the pace and the script of the movement, are used in the brain as a template for conscious thought.

Consider these facts.

An innovative program in New Jersey uses horseback riding as a form of speech therapy. Children with severe speech difficulties are taught to speak while they are riding a horse. For these children, nothing else works.

A form of yoga, that involves rhythmic breathing, is an effective remedy for obsessive compulsive disorder (OCD). OCD is a condition where extreme anxiety causes your thinking to become stuck. People with OCD painfully go over and over the same fear, day after day. The yoga works by "unsticking" the thoughts and worries.

Walking, which is an intrinsically rhythmic activity, can improve your thinking. A program of walking has been shown by medical researchers to make your thinking more efficient and flexible.

Eye movement desensitization reprocessing (EMDR) is an effective therapy for anxiety and for the treatment of the effects of trauma. The core of the technique involves rhythmic eye movement. When you undergo EMDR, the therapist teaches you to move your eyes rhythmically from side to side. As you do this, your mind is able to process thoughts and emotions that had been blocked. The rhythmic eye movement of EMDR helps your brain and your mind to think.

An innovative type of physical therapy, Feldenkrais therapy, teaches patients how to move. In his book, *Awareness Through Movement*, Feldenkrais describes the relationship between movement and thought: "working to improve movement . . . seemed to be all that was necessary to initiate unintended and nonverbal psychotherapy." In Feldenkrais therapy, people learn how to move as they learn about themselves.

Rhythmic Movement

We all want the same things. And so we all work hard. Nowadays, much of what we do is done while we are *physically inactive.* Not resting. Inactive while being mentally and emotionally stimulated. Here are some facts, to give you a picture of what is happening.

"The 'shop 'til you drop' syndrome seemed particularly active during the 1980s. . . . In the five years between 1983 and 1987, Americans purchased 51 million microwaves, 44 million washers and dryers, 85 million color televisions, 36 million refrigerators and freezers, 48 million VCRs and 23 million cordless telephones . . . 88 percent of households have a motor vehicle, and the average number of vehicles per household is two." Juliet B. Schor, *The Overworked American.*

In a way, these figures are a fantastic expression of how vibrant our culture is—when you read these figures you can almost feel the energy, the creativity and the drive.

There is just so much opportunity, so much to do. It is all quite stimulating. But it can be somewhat exhausting.

How can you tap into all of this excitement and still be at peace? How can you work as hard as you want to and still be happy? How can you be a productive, plugged-in citizen of our digital age and ever be able to relax? One way to help yourself do all of this is by using rhythmic movement. Like an essential nutrient, rhythmic movement is a daily requirement. By using a healthy amount of rhythmic movement, you can balance all of the physically inactive, mentally stimulated hours that you spend while working, driving, studying or playing on the computer. Then you will be able to rest, instead of just "dropping."

Rule #3: Use Rhythmic Movement to Help Process Your Thoughts and Feelings and Balance Mental Stimulation and Physical Inactivity

Why is this necessary? For a number of reasons, all of which are based in the way that your brain works.

The older parts of your brain, your instinctive brain, interprets the combination of physical inactivity and mental/emotional stimulation as a danger sign. To your brain, this combination means that you are in some type of trouble and that you are laying low, trying to figure out what to do. Your brain starts to send distress signals to your body. Your blood pressure rises, your muscles tense, you become vigilant and wary. Rhythmic movement reverses this brain state. It produces a calming reaction in the brain. If you are moving rhythmically, your brain senses this as a sign that everything is working well and that you can relax.

Your brain was created to think better while moving. Movement primes the pump for thinking. Movement gets the flow of your thought moving. And rhythmic movement sets the stage for processing your thoughts and emotions. It is just how your brain was created to work.

When you use rhythmic movement in a natural balance, you will find it easier to relax and to be at peace. Use rhythmic movement and you will think better—you will find that it is easier to know or to understand matters that may have been a puzzle to you.

By getting a healthy dose of rhythmic movement, you can push yourself as hard as you want or as hard as you need to and still be at peace. You will be able to rest. That can feel quite nice: working hard, accomplishing something and then resting.

What Is Your Natural Style of Rhythmic Movement?

Everyone is different. So far, you have seen how to use your personal style to help you build relationships. You have seen how to use your preferences to help you get exercise. Now extending that same idea, you can use your unique preference and attributes to pick a form of rhythmic movement that works for you.

What works for you will not work for your neighbor. While the basic bodily requirement for rhythmic movement is universal, how you get that movement is different for everybody. It can also change for you from time to time in your life. This has certainly been true in my life.

Before medical school, when I was a boy, I had always played ice hockey—as a nine-year-old Pee Wee, then in high school and in college. Anyone who has played or watched ice hockey knows that there is a beautiful rhythm to the sport. While skating, you rhythmically swing your body side to side, in graceful, swooping curves. And the action of the game sets the rhythm of skating in motion. For fifteen years, the rhythms of skating had been a part of my life. Then, because of the demands of medical school, I stopped.

As the days went by in my first year of medical school, I sped up. I talked faster. I ate faster. I walked faster. I lost my patience for normal conversation, resorting to quick one- or two-word sound bites. And I became more argumentative. With no time to hear the other person out, I would jump in, speak my mind and argue my point. Gradually, I

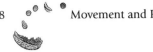

lost my physical conditioning. At the same time, I could not relax. I was wound up all of the time. Believe me, it was not pretty. I was a difficult person to be around.

Then my back went into spasms. I started to fix the problem by finding time to ski. It worked and not just because it helped me get in shape. Since I could only ski on the weekends, my physical conditioning improved to only a small degree. It worked because skiing is a rhythmic activity. It provided me with the type of rhythm my nervous system needs. It balanced all of the inactivity of my studious life with a naturally rhythmic activity.

When you ski, the slope of the hill, the spacing of the bumps, the depth of the snow all dictate the rhythm of your skiing. It is an externally applied rhythm. You either ski with the natural rhythm of the mountain, or you fall.

Years later, when my daughter was born, I really did not have the time to ski. Like everyone who is new to the complex world of being a parent, my life was pushed out of balance. I started to have trouble with my back again, in the same way—spasms. So having learned my lesson about my need for movement, I started to swim. At first, lacking natural rhythm, my swimming was an ugly sight. I flailed about in the water, inhaling water, splashing and kicking. It was a great workout, because I was so unfluid, such a nonrhythmic swimmer, I had to expend enormous amounts of energy to stay afloat. My physical conditioning improved, but that was not all that happened.

After a time, I found a natural balance of rhythmic movement. Water, because of its physical properties, demands a certain rhythm. If you swim enough, you develop a rhythm that is set by the water itself. You cannot move faster than the water allows. You cannot breathe until the right time. You must time your movements to the waves. Like skiing, swimming demands a certain external rhythm, in harmony with the properties of water.

As I swam, I settled down. Getting in shape was only part of it, as it had been with skiing. While swimming, I would get a daily fix of rhythmic motion that set a gentle pace for my nervous system. It just became easier to wait. It became easier to work in synch with the social rhythms of those around me. It became easier to relax.

These are the activities that worked for me. Unique to my physical makeup and to the circumstances in life, my rules for living include:

Paul's Rules for Movement Balance

1. *Spend at least eight hours per week in some type of rhythmic movement.*
2. *Use a whole-body, athletic activity such as skating, skiing or swimming, to meet my needs for rhythmic movement.*

That is how you create some rules for living that will help you establish a natural balance, that will help you to be as active as you want and to rest. Understand the way that you process information. Understand what is fun, interesting or exciting. Understand your unique attributes, your skills and ability. As you do, you will understand how the higher parts of your brain work in balance with the energy of your mind. Once you understand what works for you, pick a type of rhythmic movement that fits who you are.

Rule #4: Use Your Personal Style and Preferences to Pick Your Form of Rhythmic Movement

Here are some questions to guide you. Some of the questions are the same as those in the section on exercise because some forms of rhythmic movement also provide a vigorous aerobic workout.

Movement and Music

1.	Are you a good dancer?	yes	no
2.	Do you have a good sense of rhythm?	yes	no
3.	Are you musical? Do you enjoy singing or playing an instrument?	yes	no
4.	Does music help you exercise?	yes	no

If you answered yes to these questions, you may naturally be a rhythmic or musical person. In that case, rhythmic movement that is pleasurable and satisfying to you will likely involve music of some type. Music is everywhere, but in order to make this work for you, the music in your mind must guide you in a set of movements. If this works for you then your natural rules guiding a balance of movement become:

1. Use at least fifteen minutes of musical movement per day to balance inactivity.

2. The type of musical movement that works for me is (circle one):
   - playing a musical instrument
   - singing
   - dance
   - figure skating
   - _____ (other)

Athletic or Whole-Body Movement

1.	Do you enjoy activities that require whole body movement like skiing, swimming, skating, gymnastics, dance or horseback riding?	yes	no
2.	Do you feel naturally graceful or well-coordinated?	yes	no
3.	Do you find that moving your body in a coordinated way helps you to relax?	yes	no
4.	Do you find walking to be a pleasurable activity?	yes	no

A yes answer to these questions indicates that whole-body, athletic types of movement may work for you. This form of movement uses your whole body in graceful, coordinated and rhythmic motion. There are many, many ways to accomplish this type of movement: dance, yoga, ice skating, swimming, horseback riding, even walking can give you this type of movement. The list is practically endless. If this type of movement fits who you are, then this becomes one of your rules for living. Your rules would go something like this:

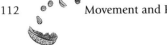

1. Spend at least eight hours per week in rhythmic movement.
2. The type of whole-body, athletic movement that works for me is (circle one):
   - dance
   - skiing
   - swimming
   - gymnastics
   - yoga
   - horseback riding
   - walking rhythmically
   - ice skating
   - _____ (other)

These are the rules that I have always followed to maintain a balance of movement and rest. Whole-body movement, ice skating, skiing or swimming to get a healthy amount of rhythmic movement has been the path that for me naturally balances movement and rest. It works for me, and if it fits your style, it can work for you.

Skilled Hand Movement

1.	Do you feel that you are "good with your hands"?	yes	no
2.	Do you enjoy painting, sculpting or pottery making?	yes	no
3.	Do you enjoy sewing, knitting or woodworking?	yes	no
4.	Do you enjoy playing a musical instrument?	yes	no
5.	Do you enjoy handwriting letters to friends and family?	yes	no

Skilled hand movement is another form of rhythmic movement that can provide a counterbalance to long periods of inactivity. Sadly, as many activities become automated, skilled hand movement is disappearing from our culture. That is too bad, since the brain pathways that allow us to have skilled hand movement are the same brain pathways that help us think. If you answered yes to any of these questions, it may mean that you can use skilled hand movement to help you to establish a healthy balance of movement in your life.

By skilled hand movement, I mean any set of hand movements that are rhythmic and which are strung together in a sequence to create something larger. Handwriting or penmanship is a good example, as are knitting or sewing or woodworking. Skilled hand work is usually creative; it involves a process of using a mind-based script—following music as you play a musical instrument is an example of a mind-based script; hand-writing a letter to a friend is another—to guide your hands in rhythmic motion. Like athletic movement and musical movement, skilled hand movement balances inactivity. An added benefit of skilled hand movement is that it can help you stay in the moment, to create something as you think. Whatever it is that you have created can be an expression of how you are thinking at the moment. This can directly help you to decrease worry and stress.

If you are good with your hands, if you enjoy skilled hand movement, then you can help yourself balance the inactivity of modern life by taking time to use skilled hand

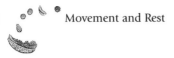

movements every day. Find time to do some woodworking. Find time to play your piano. Find time to write by hand. As you do, you will find that you are able to relax, to think more clearly and to rest. If skilled hand movement fits who you are, then your rules for living will be:

1. Spend at least fifteen minutes working skillfully with your hands for every four hours of inactivity, each day.
2. The type of skilled hand movement that works for me is (circle one):
   - writing by hand (not using a keyboard)
   - painting, sculpting or pottery making
   - woodworking
   - sewing or knitting
   - playing a musical instrument
   - drawing or drafting
   - _____ (other)

Movement and Rest Self-Test

Take this test to see if you are out of balance. If you answer yes to three or more questions, then you may have a problem with the balance of movement and rest. To improve your balance, try to incorporate the rules in this chapter as well as the tips to follow.

1. Do you prefer to drive short distances, instead of walking?	yes	no
2. If you have a choice, do you avoid physical activity?	yes	no
3. Do you have trouble getting yourself off of the couch?	yes	no
4. Are you unable to follow through on a program of exercise?	yes	no
5. Do you feel restless, edgy or uptight at the end of the day?	yes	no
6. Do you suffer with muscle tension, muscle aches or pain?	yes	no

Score _____

Tips to Balance Movement and Rest

Here is a list of tips to help you to balance movement and rest. Try some of these tips in the second week of your balance program to help yourself to get a healthy amount of movement in your life. By linking the energy and emotion of the lower centers of your brain with thought from the higher centers of your mind, movement produces a flowing and rhythmic process of thinking and feeling. Healthy movement is a natural antidote for the immobile but overstimulated style of life today.

1. Walk whenever you can. Walk to the post office, to the grocery store, to church or to your neighbor's house. Walk up stairs and down instead of using the elevator. Walk your dog, walk with your children, walk with your parents. Make up reasons to walk. Like parking at the outer reaches of the mall parking lot so you have to walk to get to the mall. Be creative! Remember that whenever you walk, you are getting healthy.

2. Vacuum the house three times a week. Really! Cleaning your home is a handy form of exercise. Research has shown that vigorous housecleaning can provide the same benefits to your health as a workout at the gym. Of course, the added benefit is that not only will you be improving your health, you will also be making your home cleaner!

3. Fill out the worksheet on page 118. It will help you to decide what type of rhythmic movement is right

for you. Then use your unique form of rhythmic movement regularly.

4. Buy a rocking chair and use it for fifteen minutes twice a day. Use this simple form of rhythmic movement to calm yourself and to help you to think. Or if you are young at heart, go for a swing on your child's swing set. The pendulum-like motion is calming to your nervous system.

5. Sing, dance or play a musical instrument. Any movement that is musical is intrinsically rhythmic. It will soothe your nervous system while engaging your mind in a healthy process. Not musically inclined? Then sing in the shower or in the car. No one will hear and you get all the benefits of singing, no matter how out of tune or out of rhythm you may be.

6. Compete at a sport. Especially true for men, competition can be one of the best motivators to help you to get enough movement in your life.

7. Breathe. Deeply, rhythmically. Breathe with your belly and not with your chest. Breathing may be the most basic pattern of rhythmic movement. By breathing deeply, with your diaphragm, about eight to twelve times a minute, you directly calm your nervous system. Now, pair breathing with another activity that includes movement and you have a terrific, balance-inducing activity. Breathe rhythmically when you sing, dance, do yoga, skate, climb, ski, swim or run. This type of combination works wonders for your mind.

8. Work with your hands. Whether you are sewing, making pottery, painting, woodworking or hand-writing notes, the process of using tools, in a patterned activity, provides you with a useful form of rhythmic movement. When you work with your hands, you activate brain pathways that help you to process your feelings and your thoughts. It can be quite relaxing. And if you make something in the process, you can take pride in the work of making something just the way you like it.

9. Move the furniture. It is surprising how satisfying this activity can be. You get the benefits of some vigorous exertion. You are able to express yourself in a usefully creative way. And you may just find a way to arrange your home that is soothing to your mind's eye. Even if you move your furniture, just for fun, then move it right back to where it was, your heart, your lungs and your mind will benefit. While your furniture is in a new location, you may even find some money that fell out of a pocket long ago!

10. Carry your child around the house, whenever you can. (Only do this if you have small children!) It is good exercise and your kids will love it.

RHYTHMIC MOVEMENT WORKSHEET
Check the box that best describes your feeling about each activity. Try to implement the most enjoyable activities into your daily life.

	NEVER ENJOYABLE	RARELY ENJOYABLE	SOMETIMES ENJOYABLE	OFTEN ENJOYABLE	USUALLY ENJOYABLE	ALWAYS ENJOYABLE
ATHLETIC OR WHOLE-BODY MOVEMENT						
Dance, ice skating or gymnastics						
Racket sports						
Martial arts						
Aerobics						
Team athletics						
Walking, hiking or climbing						
Swimming						
Skiing						
Yoga						
Horseback riding						
Other						

RHYTHMIC MOVEMENT WORKSHEET *(continued)*

MUSICAL MOVEMENT	NEVER ENJOYABLE	RARELY ENJOYABLE	SOMETIMES ENJOYABLE	OFTEN ENJOYABLE	USUALLY ENJOYABLE	ALWAYS ENJOYABLE
Playing an instrument alone						
Playing instrument as part of a group						
Singing alone						
Singing with a group						
Taking music lessons						
Acting in musical theater						
Dancing to music						
Exercising with music						
Skating with music						
Working with your hands while listening to music						
Other						

RHYTHMIC MOVEMENT WORKSHEET *(continued)*

SKILLED HAND MOVEMENT	NEVER ENJOYABLE	RARELY ENJOYABLE	SOMETIMES ENJOYABLE	OFTEN ENJOYABLE	USUALLY ENJOYABLE	ALWAYS ENJOYABLE
Painting						
Drawing or drafting						
Pottery						
Sculpting						
Sewing or knitting						
Calligraphy						
Writing by hand						
Woodworking						
Juggling						
Playing a musical instrument						
Other						

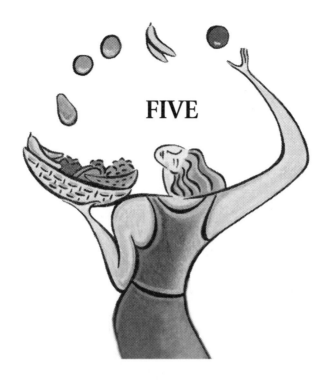

FIVE

System 3:
Living in the Present,
Living in the Past

By definition, history, and most narrative, is a
reconstructive act; it is an attempt to piece together
a large number of episodes so as to give a place
and a meaning to smaller-scale events.

Merlin Donald, *Origins of the Modern Mind*

Each person is unique. Call it your soul, your personality or your spirit, but however you label this wonderful human quality, understand that your brain was created to help you to follow a path, a story of your life that is uniquely suited to you. A path of natural balance.

What have we learned so far? That modern life, as wonderful as it may be, can upset your natural balance. That you have a personal way to reach balance, you have forms and types of movement that are unique to you; patterns of social relatedness, of human connection that are sustaining and that are unique to you.

To take the next step on your path to natural balance, it is necessary to learn how to tie it all into a story that makes sense for you. The next step on your path to balance is to understand the relationship between your moment-to-moment reactions and how these relate to your past; you must understand your experience and your unique sense of who you are. For there is a deep, fundamental relationship that exists between the way that you live in the moment and how you experience the story of your life.

Life in the Moment

How do you make sense of life? Do you struggle for meaning in the everyday blur of events? Do you find yourself reacting without a clear sense of who you are, of what you want? Or, do you find yourself unable to respond to circumstances in your life? Are you a troubled observer, wanting to take part, to jump in, but unable to? Are you inhibited by the doubts and fears that fill your mind?

The challenge is great. Never before have we humans been faced with such a pull of immediacy, the moment-to-moment demands that exist today. Here is just a partial list of day-to-day activities made possible by technologies that speed us up; technologies that provide us with abundance while at the same time placing us, moment to moment, within a rapid stream of information and events, faster than ever before:

- driving an automobile
- watching television
- surfing the Internet
- flying in an airplane
- shopping in a mall
- going to Disney World (or any theme park)
- working in a forty-story office building
- responding to cell phones and pagers
- eating at a fast food restaurant
- visiting a sick friend in the hospital
- renting a movie at a video store.

The list is practically endless. And so is the steady stream of information and events that we confront every day. It is all so immediate that modern life can overwhelm you with stimulation. It is just so easy to lose yourself in the excitement, the possibility, the *immediacy* of modern life.

This quote from David Shenk, in *Data Smog*, captures

the problem we all face: "The problem comes when the contexts begin to vanish in the sea of data."

You begin to lose context. There is just so much happening all of the time that your attention is diverted from important matters in *your* life to the excitement, the flash, the drama of life today. And the excitement may not be important to you; it is captivating because it is fast and flashy. E-mail, cell phones, airline travel, online shopping; the speed and pace grabs hold of your nervous system. It is riveting. But the information, the images and the opportunities grabbing you may not really be right for who you are.

That is how modern life and modern technologies lead you to lose the natural balance of past and present. *You lose context.*

As wonderful as life in the moment can be—spontaneous, creative, energetic and productive—it can lead you to a life out of balance. You can lose the story of your life. It can be hard to know who you are and what to do because you are so busy reacting. There is something about the way that our modern devices capture attention. The speed, the pace, the stimulation of modern life feeds into your nervous system in a way that we were not created to handle. Our ancient brains are just not designed to handle modern digital technology. Here is what Michael Dertouzous, director of the Laboratory for Computer Sciences at MIT, had to say in *Data Smog*:

"E-mail is an open duct into your central nervous system. It occupies the brain."

It occupies the brain. The steady stream of information and events that you deal with every day taps right into lower levels of your central nervous system. Absent context, your brain becomes alarmed, setting into motion a chain of events in your brain and in your mind that leads to confusion, fearfulness, self-doubt and guilt. You can end up being pulled along by events, into situations that are not right for you, while at the same time your thoughts are filled with fearfulness, confusion and self-doubt, the experience of being out of balance.

The good news is that you can make sense of life through the natural rules of balance. In the preceding chapters, you have already learned about the foundations of balance. You can make sense of how you fit; of who you are; of what is right for you. When you live with a natural balance; when you truly experience the joys of living in the moment, balanced with a sense of yourself; a confident knowledge of your past, then your life will follow a story that makes sense for you; a story unique to you; a story that flows.

Using some of the lessons you have learned in the previous two chapters; about being with people and about movement; applying these lessons in the framework of the way that your brain naturally balances the present with the past, you can find some rules to help you to a natural balance; to make sense of our fast-paced, mass media, digital world; to create a story that works for you.

Read about Melissa. Her story is about the balance of past and present.

Doing What Pleases Others

For as long as she could remember, Melissa had loved to sing; simple songs, love ballads; the rich, full-throated tones of her voice produced a sensual depth to the simple love songs she preferred. Blessed with physical beauty—black hair, deep brown eyes and a full figure—she was a natural as the lead singer for a country and western band.

And the offers came. Whenever she performed, Melissa knew that one or two musicians would approach her to sing with their band.

It began in high school. Her boyfriend convinced her to sing on stage with his band. There was no doubt it was fun for her—the music, the crowd, the attention.

She had wanted to study biology, maybe a career in teaching, so Melissa went to college. But the offers continued. She would sing three or four nights per week. The money helped too. Her dad, a schoolteacher, could not afford to pay for college. So she sang at night, attended classes in the day, and tried to get a college degree.

Years later, when she sought my help, Melissa admitted that she had never finished college. She had met a man on the plane home to visit her parents. He had a country-and-western band that played in Nashville. Lots of travel, good pay, the chance to make it big. She jumped at the opportunity, leaving college to tour with the band.

At the start, it had certainly been fun; flying around the country; seeing new places; performing before cheering crowds of people in clubs and state fairs; staying awake all night to make demonstration tapes; trying to make it big time. The lights, the music, the travel; it was exciting.

Still, in the times between performances, Melissa did not like herself. She felt false, as though her life was not her own. Not really a committed professional singer, she never felt in command of performing. She felt overwhelmed and confused by the life of a performing artist. It left her feeling like a big part of her life was missing. It did not help that she always seem to fall in love with someone from the band. The thrill of performing, the closeness of travel produced infatuations. Thrilling, but deeply disappointing relationships.

Melissa described her problem for me.

"It's not that I don't enjoy performing. I really do. When I'm singing I can forget everything. But I worry that I'm not good enough at it. I feel like a failure, since I never made it big. I feel like I failed my parents too. They wanted me to finish college, to maybe become a teacher, like my daddy. And I don't really know how to deal with all of the guys who try to hit on me. I get pulled into these relationships and the guilt just kills me. It's getting so that all I think about is what a failure I am."

Single, in her late twenties, her traveling life turned into an endless road of night clubs, county fairs and new cities; surrounded by thousands of people she didn't know and never would know, where she felt like an outsider. It had left her cynical and demoralized. "I guess I'll never be anything but a two-bit singer in a county fair band," she told me sadly.

Thankfully, the joy of performing had kept her going.

"If it weren't for my singing, I would have gotten depressed a long time ago," she told me.

But singing was not enough. It helped her to feel better for *a time but it was not enough. Melissa's life was out of balance. She sang so well, so easily, with a natural charm, that her singing worked against her. In the excitement of the crowds, the music, the romance, her singing actually worked to keep her in the moment, with no clear sense of herself. Melissa lost the story of her life; she lost touch with who she was, what she valued and what she really wanted for herself.*

As we talked, Melissa got in touch with a side of herself that she had all but forgotten. She recalled the hours she had spent in the woods behind her house, collecting bugs, watching squirrels, picking up interesting plants. She and her father had set up a glass case in the basement for her treasures. There she spent countless hours arranging her bugs and flowers; drawing and categorizing her specimens, then looking in her natural history encyclopedia to find the exact species she had collected. She had dreamed of being a veterinarian or a scientist, researching the mysteries of the animals and plants she loved.

Curious by nature, with an eye for detail, every night at dinner she told her mother and her father about her wonderful discoveries. Her parents were charmed by her intelligent enthusiasm, and it showed. "I loved it," she told me, "I used to feel so good that they liked listening to me talk about my discoveries. I had forgotten this, but my daddy used to call me his 'little scientist' because of the way I had filled my glass case and my room with bugs, plants and other creatures."

From her story, we developed a list of the activities that came naturally to her.

Melissa's natural activities

- teaching
- singing
- researching nature
- organizing or cataloguing
- talking about ideas and discoveries

"I can't see how this all fits," she told me, "I've never been able to make sense of what I like." So we set a plan to meet and talk; our subject would be her story, to figure out how the pieces of her life fit together.

It occurred to Melissa, that she had been drawn into the entertainment world so quickly, that she had never had a chance to think these things through.

"My daddy really wanted me to finish college. We had a big fight when I told him I was quitting to sing with a band. We stopped talking for a long time. Until then, I had always gone to him for advice. But you know, he never wanted me to sing. I think he was afraid of what would happen."

It was true. Worried about Melissa, that her good looks and beautiful voice would take her away, he had always been critical about her singing. He had made her feel so badly, that in defiance, she gave up on her career in biology. Being a singer was just too much fun for her to put up with the years of study she would need to be a veterinarian.

As we talked, Melissa started to understand her story and how she could put it all together. She did not have to be a singer or a scientist; she could be both. In balance. All along, she had known that her singing was the way that she enjoyed being with people. It was not a career. It was pleasure. On the other hand, she had a passion for natural science, for creatures of all kinds. Exploring nature, in the field and in the world of ideas, was what she wanted. She had a passion to find out how it all related; how it all worked.

As she got in touch with her story, Melissa began to see how she could leave the entertainment world. She knew she should go back to school. But before doing so, Melissa had to train herself; she had to find a way to keep from getting drawn into the momentary excitement of the entertainment world. She did this in two ways. She found a reading group; women, like herself, interested in a career in the sciences. Sitting with the group helped her to be more certain of her identity as a student of the natural sciences. Then, she purchased a small diary. In it she wrote her ideas about singing; that it was for entertainment, that it was okay to sing and enjoy herself without having it take over her life, that it was a joyful hobby, a form of expression, a complement to her more serious side.

She kept her diary with her. And when the moment struck, she would read what she wrote. It helped her to enjoy her singing, while placing it in the larger context of her life. And she developed a deeper understanding of who she was; more confident in herself, she left the band to attend college near home. Her goal: to become a veterinarian; to use her natural interest in science and her natural ability to observe, to organize and to categorize.

"I patched things up with my daddy. After all these years, he's accepted my singing. Want to know an amazing thing? He found a local band, you know, a weekend and wedding-type band for me to sing with. And I got a job, at the natural history museum, to help pay for school. I'll be helping with the collections and giving tours."

Melissa restored balance in her life by discovering the natural balance of past and present; by learning about her skills, about the activities that for her, were natural; a part of who she is. Then, through conversations with me and later with her dad, she learned how to create a story that fit who she is.

How Does Your Brain Balance Past and Present?

As you live and grow, as the experiences of your life interact with your natural ability, you develop a set of behaviors that you can reliably employ to carry out your day-to-day activities. A personal repertoire of behaviors. A set of routines. Let's call these behaviors and routines your *tools*. The idea of a toolbox, filled with a set of your own personal life tools, collected over a lifetime of experience, is a helpful image, a useful symbol for a fundamental aspect of brain function. In Melissa's story, her tools have been listed for you to see. They are her skills, but they really are the *tools* of behavior that she used to conduct her life.

Your brain is wired to react to events, in the moment, by activating preset behavioral routines—your personal tools. It is a wonderfully efficient system. Before you know it, somewhat automatically, as you confront a life event, your brain picks a tool and uses it—to handle the circumstances for you. Automatic, in part, as an inborn survival mechanism, some tools, some behavioral routines, are so important for survival that your brain activates them in a flash. You can be into a behavioral response before you know it. *Before you know it.* Your brain, so attuned to survival, can pick and use a tool to deal with a situation before you have had a chance to reflect.

Researchers have confirmed this notion. Cognitive researchers have shown that one way the brain creates a behavior for you is by using preset, cognitive- or thought-based patterns, called schemas, that are sequential and predictable for a given person. Neurological researchers have found the brain pathways for these schemas, made up of nerves linking lower centers and higher centers in the brain. These brain pathways are really neural circuits. When stimulated into action, the circuits produce the preset behavioral responses that we are calling your tools. A neurosurgeon can actually touch a part of your brain with an electrode and produce a fully formed behavior, like singing, throwing a ball or having a conversation, out of thin air.

As a child, this is an automatic and unthinking process. Gradually, as you grow and learn, you begin to exert some conscious control over the process of tool selection and tool use. You develop a sense of what to do, based on who you are, what you value and where you have been in life. That is a good thing. Imagine, for a moment, a world where you only reacted, without thinking; a world without context, where your actions and responses were based entirely on the contingencies of the moment. This is not the world of human life. It is an instinctive world of brute survival, a world that lacks the basic human qualities we prize—kindness, loyalty, love, trust, empathy, altruism. Fortunately, the wisdom of creation has given us a brain and mind which, in its natural mode of functioning, can produce a balanced, rhythmic and harmonious behavior that is so essentially human.

Recall that your brain always works in balance. The instinctive stimulation, the activation, from the lower centers in your brain, that activates your behavioral tools is balanced by thought from higher centers in the brain. Spontaneous action is balanced by memory, by learning and by experience. As you live, you remember.

Your brain was created to notice the results produced by your different behavioral tools, to size up what works and what doesn't, and to orchestrate and organize how and when you use your tools. By noticing how you do, by remembering the results of your actions, by comparing the effects of your actions, your brain develops a story or narrative to guide you in the selection and use of your tools. Your brain balances in-the-moment living by naturally creating a personal story of how things work for you.

As your story develops, you are able to *read* your personal story. Then you can decide if you like it, if it works for you, if your actions are helpful to you and to those you love. By reading your own personal story, you can learn and grow, developing tools that you value, discarding others that do not work.

That is how you live in balance. That is the path you can follow to balance the present of life-in-the-moment with the past of your own personal story.

Here is a story about Hal and how he learned to read the story of his life.

Burned Out by Work

Hal consulted me because he was drinking too much. Every night after work, he stopped at the liquor store. He bought a nip of bourbon for the road and two six-packs of beer, which he drank while he ate frozen pizza and watched television.

"I'm just so burned out by work, Doc, it's all I can do," he told me.

Hal worked hard. Starting as a technician in the testing lab, he had worked his way into a management position. That is when his troubles began.

"I'm reacting all day. E-mails from everyone. My boss tells me what to do. The guys on my team complain. Our customers call and make demands. I just put out one fire after another." The work had consumed his life. Pulled from one insistent demand to another, Hal worked eighty hour per week. There was no time left over for him to think.

"The drinking started about two years ago. We had a union problem at work. And I used to be a union guy, so I took it on as a personal cause. I would come home from work and talk to my guys by e-mail, you know, to settle them down. While I was doing it, I drank beer. It was a time thing. The beer was in the fridge, easy to get and it tasted good going down. Then it became a habit."

This was not the life that Hal wanted. He enjoyed designing circuits for computer chips. But he spent most of his time managing people. Yet he was lonely. He was too tired to socialize after work. And his people contact was limited to his boss, his clients and to the people he supervised. At the end of the day, he drank. He became negative and self-critical. He began to doubt that he could do his job. Hal suffered with a feeling that he had made a terrible mess out of his life.

Hal's life was out of balance. He had lost his bearings, lost touch with his story. Life, for him, was a burnout—one emergency after another; one demand after another with no room for him and his interests. Unable to quiet his doubts and self-criticism any other way, he drank. It was all that he had.

To help him find his path, I gave Hal an assignment that we worked on together. The assignment was to list four activities that he liked and that he felt he was good at:

Hal's list
1. Designing electronic devices
2. Bicycling
3. Playing softball
4. Fixing things

We turned this list into Hal's first rule for living. Hal learned how to balance the past and present by using his tools. Putting this another way, Hal learned how to stay calm, focused and happy by using his natural skills, abilities and interests.

Hal's tool kit:
- work as a design engineer
- work as part of a team

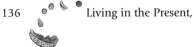

- spend time riding a bike or working out to keep fit
- relax by doing projects at home

Whenever he was feeling hassled, harried, confused and overwhelmed by the moment-to-moment demands of his life, Hal made sure to spend some time using the tools in his behavioral tool kit. These activities came naturally to him. Hal felt an easy rhythm, a natural flow and a sense that things would work out fine when he was using his behavioral tools. His confidence returned as he spent time engaged in activities that he felt good about, activities that fit him well. He could make sense of his life as he did these things. Less stressed, he began to cut down on his drinking, spending time after work bicycling or working on interesting projects at home.

As he used his tools, as he worked with the repertoire of behaviors that fit, he began to feel better. Hal had a better sense of how his life could work for him, a better sense of how to fit the pieces together.

Hal could see that he was spending most of his day in an activity that he did not feel suited for. Working with people problems was not something he liked, and he did not feel that he was good at it. As he went through his day, each situation that he dealt with made him feel frustration and a sense of failure.

"I never realized it before. I just started doing it. The next thing you know, my whole job is dealing with people, and I'm feeling burned out and stupid."

He had been such a hard worker, so capable, that Hal had been promoted into a position that did not fit who he was. Still, he wasn't sure what to do. He couldn't yet make sense of how to create a story. Then he met Claudia. She was a member of his bicycle club. They were like two peas in a pod: the same interests, the same values, the same way of looking at life.

This led Hal to his next rule for living: Talk with Claudia to help me understand and accept my own story.

Through the loving support provided by Claudia, Hal was able talk openly and to discover his real story.

"Claudia and I talk all the time, Doc. We've talked about these tools that you say I should use. Claudia thinks you're right. She thinks I need to get out of management at work. She says I'll do better working with a design team, kind of like being on a softball team. But I'm not sure how to pull this off."

So we worked on a way for Hal to read his story—the one that Claudia had helped him to understand. This was Hal's next rule for living—become good at reading his story. Since Hal's problem was that he was flooded by moment-to-moment crises at work, people problems and management work, it was hard for Hal to remember his story. It was hard for him to make choices based on his story. We came up with a system to help him remember his priorities. Hal got some three-by-five cards and on each card, Hal wrote a phrase that reminded him of what he liked to do. Here is what Hal wrote:

- Focus on the engineering problem, not on the people
- You are part of a team; ask for their help.
- Work is just work; save time for your life.

- You can always try to work things out later.
- Try to get back to your circuits.

Each time Hal found himself becoming drawn into the moment, he pulled out his three-by-five cards to remind himself of his story, of who he was and how he felt good about himself. As he did this, he became more patient, better at delegation. He found that he could ask members of his team to solve some of the problems for him. There was more time for him to focus on the engineering problems faced by his team.

He gained confidence in himself. And as he did, his life really began to change. More open to possibilities that fit for him, his relationship with Claudia grew. He and Claudia married. They bought a fixer-upper of a home, closer to work. He and Claudia worked on it together. It was a joint project, a satisfying blend of fixing what was broken to create a home. By getting rid of his lengthy and stressful commute, Hal was able to ride his bicycle to and from work. The days of stopping at the liquor store on the way home were over.

As Hal lived within the story of his life, he felt better. His drinking stopped. He began to feel balance.

Here we are trying to make sense of life in a digital world, using our ancient, tribal brains. What a time it is. The challenge to you is to find a way to live in a rapid-paced, stimulating world of immediacy, while staying true to who you are. You can. But first, let's understand the problem in a little more depth.

Your very human brain developed over millions of years

to function in balance with a world that was slow and predictable. The same two hundred people, the same ten square miles of geography, the same climate and the same daily tasks. As you might imagine, it was not difficult for our ancestors to make sense of life. The day-to-day story was the same as it had been for tens of thousands of years. You would raise children, find food, avoid danger, make whatever implements you needed for life. You would see the members of your village every day. Life was clear, simple and predictable, a match for your repertoire of behaviors, there was a tight match between the needs of your life and your personal set of behavioral tools.

And then all of this changed in the last two hundred years. It is still changing at an ever-faster pace. Instead of facing a simple and predictable set of circumstances, each day you are flooded, quite literally flooded, with information, ideas, possibilities and people. Instead of dealing with the slow evolution of tribal matters, you are flooded by matters that change minute by minute. And it all comes to your attention in a gripping and stimulating way: as you drive your car, fly in an airplane, watch your television, listen to your cell phone, use your computer or shop at the mall.

Here is the problem. Digital-age technologies grab ahold of your ancient brain in a way that can unbalance your mind. It can pull you into a moment-by-moment, sound-byte style of living that few of us, if anyone, can deal with very well. Modern, electronic, digital technologies get right into the lower centers of your brain, lighting it up like a Christmas tree. And so you react. Of course you do; your brain is programmed to do so. You become pulled into the moment. It may be exciting. It may be productive. It may be fun. But it may not fit.

When you spend your day flooded with digital-age stimulation, your brain becomes alarmed and you can become stressed.

What's more, there is just so much information to deal with that you begin to feel overwhelmed and incompetent. As though you are a faceless number, a simple cog in a huge confusing machine, instead of a unique person. As though you can't comprehend your situation fully, or are unable to finish a task. As though you will fail to understand or to master whatever it is that is coming at you. You can, paradoxically, become lost in the past—lost in failure, bad feeling and regret. That is what happens when you live with a flood of immediacy; your brain, living in a constant state of alarm, tells you that things are not right.

If you spend your time watching Julia Roberts in the movies, how on earth can you ever feel attractive enough to feel good about yourself? Your ancient brain reacts with envy. If all day long, you hear about Bill Gates and his billions, how can you be satisfied with your job? Your ancient brain will tell you that you have failed. If all day long you are flooded with stock quotes, weather information, drama, jokes, opinions and "breaking news," your ancient brain tells you that disaster is about to strike. How on earth can you ever figure out what to do?

Instead, your overstimulated brain operates out of balance. And you end up feeling overwhelmed, as though you are failing, as though bad things are about to happen—even when your life, by all measures, is a success. The answer is balance.

You have seen how it worked for Melissa and for Hal. It can work for you. Let's develop the rules that will help you balance the excitement and richness of the present, with your story and experiences from your past that tell you how to make it all fit.

Picking Your Tools

Recall, if you will, what we learned in the previous chapters on relationships and movement. Here are the main points:

1. You have a unique and natural way of being with people that comes from the information-processing style, hard-wired from birth into your brain. When you relate to others, in your natural style, it feels right. It will flow and feel comfortable. And it will help you form the kind of close relationships that are healthy and sustaining.

2. Having five or more close relationships is good for your health. Close relationships help you maintain balance in all areas of your life, body and mind.

3. You have a unique and natural style of movement based on your interests, your makeup and your ability. Using your preferred style of movement helps you get enough healthy exercise.

4. Your body and mind function more effectively when you have enough rhythmic movement in your life. Rhythmic movement provides the music for your mind, helping you process your thoughts and your feelings. Rhythmic movement is the antidote to the mentally stimulated but physically inactive lifestyle of today. There is a style of rhythmic movement that is right for you.

You can use these points of balance to develop your tools for a healthy balance of past and present; you can develop the skills, activities and behaviors that are natural for you, the tools that you can draw on to be comfortably active in the moment.

Here's how you do it. Let's start with the way that you naturally prefer to be with people. In chapter three, you learned about your natural style of information processing. Your natural style will fall into one of the following categories:

Verbal

Dramatic/Emotional

Visual/Mechanical

Intellectual/Professional

Athletic

Musical

Following your natural style of information processing, you can develop activities that will help you to form and sustain meaningful relationships with people you care about. For example, if you understand and enjoy the world of music, then relating to people by sharing musical activities makes sense for you. The people activities that are based on your natural style of information processing will be fun, satisfying and rewarding to you.

List your preferred people activities here:

_____

_____

_____

You will use these activities later, to develop your toolbox of behavioral tools.

Next, let's focus on movement. In chapter four, you answered a questionnaire that helped you to understand what your natural preferences are in regards to exercise. Your preferences are important because exercising is easier to accomplish when you feel excited, rewarded or engaged by certain forms of movement. In broad terms, your natural preference for vigorous movement or exercise will probably fit into one or more of the following categories:

_____ activities that require eye-hand coordination
_____ activities that require whole body movement
_____ exercising with others
_____ exercising in a class, such as dance,
        aerobics or martial arts
_____ high stimulation exercise such as rock climbing,
        skiing or mountain biking
_____ activities that involve competition

____ endurance activities like running,
    swimming or triathlon
____ exercising with music
____ exercise that has another purpose like gardening
    or home construction

Following your natural preferences for vigorous movement will help you to develop healthy and sustainable exercise habits. For example, if endurance activities are interesting to you, then participating in triathalons may be a good way for you to include exercise in your life. Alternately, if you enjoy activities that require eye-hand coordination, then playing tennis, volleyball or racketball may help you to include exercise in your life.

The forms of vigorous movement that are appealing to you can then become part of your toolbox of reliable behavioral tools.

List your exercise preferences here:

_____

_____

_____

The last type of activity to think about in developing your tools is rhythmic movement, movement that follows a rhythmic, melodic or musical pattern. Movement that has a timing to it, a pace and a flow. Movement that has a musical pattern. Movement that follows a flowing script. This type of movement naturally calms you. It naturally helps your brain to process your emotions and your thoughts.

In chapter 4, you answered some questions that helped you to understand what type of rhythmic movement you prefer. Your preference will probably fall into one of the following categories:

____ musical movement such as singing, dance or figure skating
____ whole-body movement such as swimming, skiing, dance or horseback riding
____ skilled hand movement such as painting, sewing or woodworking

Thinking about your preferred type of rhythmic movement, then list preferences here:

_____

_____

_____

These rhythmic movement activities become part of your behavioral toolbox. Since rhythmic movement has a calming effect on your nervous system, the behavioral tools that are derived from your preferences for rhythmic movement are particularly important. These tools help you to calm and soothe yourself whenever the frenetic pace of today's information age causes you to become uptight, worried and frazzled.

You may recall, from Hal's story, that rule number one

for the balance of past and present is to *pick your tools. Your tools* are activities, behaviors really, that happen naturally for you. Your tools are your behavioral routines, to be used in a somewhat automatic fashion, as a natural and healthy way of being in the moment; they are a way of being that is in balance with your nervous system and with who you are.

Review the lists you have created. From these lists, you should be able to create a list of tools made up of combinations of your preferred styles of activity.

This activity leads you to your first rule for the balance of past and present. From the lists you have created you can do the following: *Understand and accept your natural skills.* I call this picking your tools.

Rule #1: Pick Your Tools

_____

_____

_____

_____

_____

_____

In the two stories in this chapter, there are good examples of picking tools. Melissa found that organizing or cataloguing were pleasing activities for her. She used this insight as the basis for going back to school and finding a job in a museum. Hal found that he preferred to work with people as a member of a team, rather than as a solitary leader. This insight helped him reorganize his work group to function as a team which then allowed him to delegate tasks and problems while freeing up time for the design work he loved.

There are as many behavioral tools as there are people. Discovering yours does not have to be confusing. Simply pay attention to your natural style of being with people and your natural style of activity, then using some insight, turn these preferences into reliable behavioral tools that you can use. How you use your tools to create a flowing and harmonious story for your life is the focus of the next natural rule of balance.

Create a Story for Your Life

About 200,000 years ago, when our ancestors began to live together in villages and tribes, when members of a village began to perform different day-to-day roles to support each other, when humans began to learn to use tools, a fundamental change occurred in the functioning of the human brain. The human brain grew larger—much larger—from an average size of 700 cc to the present size of 1400 cc. This is roughly equivalent to the change in size from a large grapefruit to the size of a cabbage. At the same time, language developed. Human beings learned to talk. And we learned how to tell stories, to create a narrative. It happened naturally. As the human world grew in complexity, the human brain developed a capacity to tell a story that explained how all of the pieces fit.

Researchers agree this change happened so that humans could explain how life worked—to provide a set of instructions, to reliably guide behavior in the ancient villages; to allow human beings to be social and to depend on one another. Our brains developed in balance with the physical skills we are given, in harmony with the needs, the interests and the experience of the people we care about. The change is what truly makes us human.

The ability to tell a story is nature's way of providing you with a set of operating instructions for the complex machine that is your body and mind. But here is the catch. Nature provided this wonderful ability so that you could be social, part of a group of interdependent human beings. Learning your own story, and how you fit, is a process of social learning. You learn your own story through the help of others. To create a unique and satisfying personal story, one that fits your tool set, you will need the help of others, to observe, to guide and to support.

Throughout time people have learned their personal story through the help of others. That is what we all do as parents, for our children. That is why we humans have always learned skills and crafts by becoming an apprentice to someone else. That is why mentors, counselors, coaches and priests are all so important in human history. That is why we gather together in schools and universities, so that we can learn from wise, experienced and expert people how to create a personal story.

Some of that essential function is being lost. Each time a teacher is replaced by an online course, some of that is lost. Each time an in-person supervising relationship is replaced by e-mail, some of that is lost. Each time you move away from your extended family and close friends, some of that is lost. Each time you replace conversation with television, some of that is lost.

And so we are losing our way. But you can put this key function back into your life. This leads to the next rule of balance for past and present: the rule for living about creating your own story.

Rule #2: Balance the Present by Creating a Story for Your Life

By creating a set of tools, you have found the skills and the activities that help you to function effectively in the present. Now you need a story that tells you how, when and where to use your tools. Call it your identity; call it your profession; call it your area of expertise; no matter how you think about your guiding principles, you are really using an internal narrative or story of who you are.

You find your story through the help of others, by finding a person, or a group of people who are supportive, who are wise with experience, who can tell you what they see and who can guide you. Since this is a time-honored human function, the resources are plentiful. All that is necessary is for you to pick one that works for you.

Here are some typical methods of learning your own story:

- in counseling or therapy
- by attending church

- by becoming an apprentice to a skilled practitioner (this is what doctors do in training, when we are interns and residents)
- by attending school
- by working with a coach or tutor
- by talking with the elder members of your family
- by joining an interest group

The point is not simply to attend these activities. The relationship you create will help you find context. It will help you to create a story or a plan for you to use your natural behavioral tools, your skills, abilities and interests in a continuous flow that fits who you are. Learn from the experience and guidance of others to create a story of your life that tells you how to use your personal tools.

The Balance of Past and Present: Reading Your Own Story

Once you have defined your tool set, once you have created a personal story, the next task is to become good at reading and applying your own story. Now, more than ever, that is a challenge. All of the instantaneous stimulation, all of the possibilities, all of the excitement in your life can overwhelm you; it can flood your awareness and cause you to lose your way. Modern life can cause you to lose touch with your own story. And when it does, you can be burdened with the past, with a sense that somehow you have failed. In fact, the images and sounds of today can confuse your thinking by design. The mass media culture is created to replace your personal story with the story from the media. The mass media tells you to eat, to shop, to spend, to feel drama and excitement, to put aside whatever you are doing to be entertained. The message is follow our story not yours. It is powerful; it is everywhere, and it is confusing.

But there is an answer. It lies in the next rule of balance: become good at reading your own story. To live with a healthy balance of past and present, you must learn to read your own story, to be true to yourself and to follow a script that makes sense for who you are and where you are in life. It is not enough to simply learn about yourself. To live in balance you must follow your own story, living within the helpful structure of your identity.

There is quite a lot that you can do. In fact, skilled researchers have provided us with clear guidance about ways you can become good at telling your own story. The researchers, called cognitive neuroscientists, have studied the mind, developing techniques to help you read and apply your story.

It is all about memory, the kind of memory that keeps running tabs on your experience. Not the memory for facts and figures. Not the memory for names. But rather, the memory of processes; the memory of how you do things, especially, the memory of how you relate to people. For that is how we survive. By remembering the processes that work. By remembering who you can rely on.

You do this by recalling key phrases, key images and key connections that represent the processes that work. It is like remembering elements of a story. Or it can be compared to remembering landmarks on a journey.

Depending on your natural style of information processing, these reminders can be words, pictures, movements, emotions, ideas, objects or a combination of each. The technique involves creating a set of memories that recalls a process with a positive outcome. Here are some examples. Recall, if you will, that Hal used three-by-five cards with helpful phrases written on them to remind him of his story: that he worked better in a team, that he was happier focused on engineering work and that work is only a part of his life, not all of it. Melissa used a diary to remind her that she loved science and the study of plants and animals. She used her diary to remind her that singing was a pleasure, enjoyment and not a lifestyle. One woman I know, an artist, used a collection of pictures, a collage, to keep her on track and to remind her of her story: that the joy and beauty in her life came from her art, that she could feel good about her creative processes and that the troubles she was having with her husband would work out, if she stayed true to her artistic vision.

And then there is my friend Bill, an engineer. Whenever I met Bill, he was always working on calculations and diagrams. It is just his way of orienting himself to who he is and what is important; it helps him to remember his story. He came to me for help with a family problem. Before every session, I would find him writing away in his notebook. Here is what he told me:

"I'm an engineer, you see. It's what got me where I am. I may have problems with my wife and kids that I'm a bit puzzled about, but I'm not puzzled about my work. I work on my calculations. Draw them up, try to get the thing to work right. Engineering is what I do. It's what I feel good about. I figure that I'll get you to help me with the stuff that gives me trouble."

Working on his engineering calculations and diagrams is Bill's way of becoming good at telling his story. Indeed, the confidence he felt in his engineering helped him work through the problems with his family.

Rule #3: Become Good at Reading Your Own Story

Use landmarks or cues that remind you of the story you have created for your life. Your story is made up of your tools, the behaviors that come naturally to you, used in a process that feels right, a process that you value—your story.

Here are some ideas for cues:

- a collection of key phrases written on cue cards (like Hal)
- a diary (like Melissa)
- pictures carried with you
- positive or affirming phrases that you remember or repeat at key moments
- music that guides the telling of your story
- movement, like working with tools or sewing
- praying

The possibilities are endless, as long as the cues you choose remind you of your story, telling you something fundamental about the key processes of your life. As long as the cues can clearly and strongly direct you away from moment-to-moment stimulation, on to your own personal story, then they will work. Your cues will activate your mind to create a narrative, a guiding vision, a story of who you are.

To illustrate how this all works in real life, listen to a brief story of how I developed my professional career. As you can tell from the earlier chapters, my life seems to flow better when I am involved with the world of ideas and with the world of athletics. If that sounds a bit confusing, then you can understand how I felt early in my career. There I was, plowing ahead through psychiatry training, which was, and still very much is, a world of ideas. And at the same time, I was a dyed-in-the-wool jock. What confusion. On the one hand, my supervisors were training me to listen, to observe, to think and to defer all to the needs of my patients. On the other hand, I couldn't wait to elbow my opponent aside on the squash court, or to bust a few good runs down the ski hill or to destroy my opponent with a killer drive, winning a few bucks, at my Saturday golf match. And the busier I became, the more my competitive instincts took over— moving fast, jostling for position, taking a shot when I had an opening. As you might imagine, this type of behavior did not work very well in my work as a psychiatrist.

I recall one supervisor in particular, a psychoanalyst, telling me in exasperation, "Paul, you've got to learn to wait before you give advice. Sit and wait for what your patient needs to say."

I was perplexed. I could see that being a good doctor

means being a good listener. It means being able to patiently wait, gathering history, providing support when it is needed, acting only when it was best for my patient. It is probably an understatement to say that this was not necessarily a good fit for who I was. I felt out of balance. Pulled by the excitement of the moment to a competitive pattern of behavior, I began to feel that perhaps I was a bad fit for a life as a psychiatrist.

Then I met Edward (Ned) Hallowell, M.D. He was a supervising psychiatrist at Harvard Medical School. Now, of course, he is a renowned author, an expert in the field of psychiatry.

I'll never forget the day I went to his office for supervision. He was sitting back in a chair, feet up on his desk, listening to music, looking for all the world like he was having a great time, comfortable within the confusing world of being a psychiatrist. I was intrigued and for good reason. Like myself, Ned is an athlete. And he had been able to successfully integrate movement and sports into his identity as a psychiatrist. He took an interest in me and invited me to play squash. He had a good sense that it would be easier to talk on the squash court than it would be in his office.

In life, and certainly in medicine, everyone needs a guide. Ned became mine. As we played squash, and under his subtle guidance, I honestly looked at who I was. I developed a better idea of my own skills, abilities and interests. I developed the tools in my behavioral tool kit—tools that I could use in life.

Paul's tool kit:

- Stay active in athletics. Socialize through the world of sport.
- Work in a team setting.
- Connect to the world of ideas.
- Write for pleasure as well as for work.
- Work as a professional.

Over time, we became friends. It is hard to describe the exact nature of the relationship. We talk like colleagues. We compete with each other in sports, sometimes with furious intensity. And I always look to Ned for advice. He is just the sort of guide that fits my life. I look to him for advice, for guidance, for encouragement and, most importantly, for an honest perspective on my story. Through talking, while playing squash with Ned, I have been able to develop a sensible story for my life. Athletics, long the mainstay of my life—athletic activity resonates in deep harmony with who I am—fits in my adult life as a pathway to social activity, to fun and health. But athletics is only a part of who I am. To achieve balance, my story has to include the world of ideas, and it must include acting on behalf of others, as a professional. What started out as a confusing and conflicting set of expectations—conflicts that were pushed aside when I became busy with life, pulled into the excitement of the moment, conflicts that were replaced by my familiar competitive instincts—turned into a story for me that fit. Here it is.

Paul's Guiding Story

Work as a professional, with a team of like-minded people, toward a common goal. That goal, the form of treatment administered, must be positive, active, encouraging and problem-oriented.

Write to stay involved with the world of ideas, to generate fresh perspectives, to share information, and to help with self-perspective and thinking through situations in my life.

Socialize with friends and family through the world of athletics. Stay involved with sports as a path to relaxation, social enjoyment and physical health.

How I Learned to Read My Story

It was easier for me to formulate a story than it was to become adept at reading my own story. Whenever I was drawn to the moment, by a phone call, a page or an e-mail, or by a middle-of-the-night emergency, out came my competitive instincts. In the excitement of the moment, I forgot about my behavioral tools; I forgot about the story I had worked out. My brain, my mind and I would all move instinctively, competitively, in a quick and reactive fashion. It was not helpful, and it left me feeling badly.

The answer came to me through my discussions with Ned. We were playing squash one day, while discussing a difficult situation with a psychologist who worked with us. Up came my usual instinctive response. It went something like, "He can do it my way, or I'll bypass him and just do it myself." Ned, in his usual insightful and subtle way said: "Why don't you talk to Christine? Get her take on the matter. See what she might do." Christine is our office manager, the best people person imaginable. She is someone who unfailingly knows the right thing to do for people.

And the light bulb went off in my head. I recalled my years of playing ice hockey, on a team. Trying to go it alone on the ice rink never worked. You had to pass the puck, work with your teammates, talk with each other to figure out the next play. That was what I needed to do. I needed to talk with my team whenever I felt my old go-it-alone competitive instincts rising; talking to people on my team would help me read my story, to use my behavior tools in the way that I wanted, to not become lost in the moment but to stay in a balance of my present and the correct and healthy guidance of my past. That was how I learned to read my own story. It led to the creation of my third rule for balancing past and present.

My Rules for Becoming Good at Reading My Story

1. *Always talk to my team when under pressure, to keep me on track with my story.*

That was my path to the balance of past and present. For me, talking with members of my team reminds me of the processes and paths of my story. It helps me to pull out of the moment, to activate my behavioral tools and to move in harmony with who I really am. That was the path I followed to develop my career, finding a way to use my tools in harmony with who I am. Hopefully, my story has given you a picture of how you can achieve balance, too.

Living in the Present, Living in the Past Self-Test

Take this test to see if you are out of balance. If you answer yes to three or more questions, then you may have a problem with the balance of past and present. To improve your balance, try to incorporate the rules in this chapter as well as the tips to follow.

1. Do you often find yourself reacting to events without a plan and without time to think?	yes	no
2. Do you often find yourself feeling overwhelmed and incompetent even when things turn out okay?	yes	no
3. Do you sometimes feel stumped by a problem in your life because you can't decide what steps to take?	yes	no
4. Do you often find yourself engaged in an activity when you had not intended to get involved?	yes	no
5. Do you sometimes feel that your life has lost its meaning or that your goals no longer make sense?	yes	no

Score_____

Tips to Balance the Past and Present

Here is a list of tips to help you to balance your moment-to-moment reactions with a strong sense of your past, your experience and your unique sense of who you are. For there is a deep, fundamental relationship that exists between the way that you live in the moment and how you experience the story of your life.

Try some of these tips in the third week of your balance program. By doing so, you will be taking the next steps on your path to balance. Understand the relationship between your moment-to-moment reactions and how these relate to your past, your experience and to your personal story.

1. Ask someone who cares about you to name three activities that you are good at. Often, others are better at identifying your skills than you may be yourself. These three activities may be part of your behavioral tool kit.

2. Think about someone who makes you smile. Then, figure out why. If the reason for your smile is an activity you engage in with that person, then you have another clue about your behavioral tools. That activity may be a tool you can use to effectively relate to others.

3. Take out a photo album and pick out the pictures where you are smiling and happy. Think about what you were doing at that time. Consider including these events, activities or occasions as a regular part of your life. Or better yet, set your life on a path that leads you to these happy occasions. For example, if there is a picture of you smiling with some co-workers, then perhaps the work project

from that time is, in some way, important to you.

4. Leave time to do what you enjoy (so long as it safe, legal and moral). The activities you enjoy are usually based on your natural skills. These are part of your tools.

5. Make a habit of seeking advice from someone you trust. Ask for advice about what you should do or how you might best handle a particular situation. This will help you to learn your own story.

6. Seek out people from your past. Get their take on how you handled yourself successfully, in that past. Ask them, what worked well, what didn't, and what could you have done differently. This will help you to get a sense of who you are and what your skill may be over time. This is your story.

7. Look for external recognition of your activities. Whether it is a professional license such as a law degree, or a brown belt at karate class, or even following a recipe from your favorite cookbook, meeting the standards of a recognized group can be a satisfying way to create a story. When you follow the principles and practices of an organized group you are really following a story that fits for you. Such principles and practices are a good way to help yourself from being lost in the moment.

8. Carry a good luck charm. It could be a favorite picture, a coin that has a special meaning, a particular piece of jewelry, or some meaningful words

written on a small piece of paper. All that matters is that your good luck charm reminds you of an important element of who you are. The luck that this unique belonging brings to you is the luck that comes from staying in balance with your own story.

9. Make a habit of telling your story to someone you care about. Tell them how and why you are doing what you do. Share your plans, your ideas and your goals. Describe what went right and what went wrong. As you tell your story, you will be creating an active memory of who you are and who you want to be.

10. Pray. Whether you are religious or not, silently repeating a prayer is a way of telling your story. A helpful prayer effectively captures an element of who you are, and of how you want to behave. Prayer can be an effective tool for reading your own story, especially when the going gets tough.

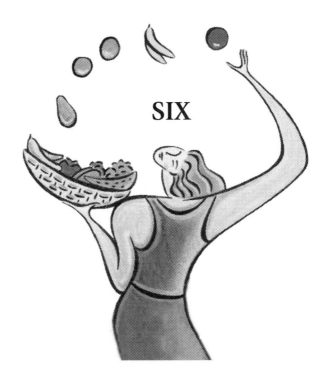

SIX

System 4:
The Energy of
Your Appetites

It's about passion, sensual pleasure, deep pulls, lust, fears, yearning hungers. It's about needs so strong they're crippling.

Caroline Knapp, *Drinking: A Love Story*

The Abundance of Life Today

In today's world, you must create your own appetite and energy balance. Why? Because never before have so many of us had so many resources at our disposal. Never before have so many of us been so able to gather food, to find a mate, to experience the pleasures of drink with so little effort. Unlike any other time in human history, you can consume without fear, you can consume without worry about when or where you will be able to consume again. In fact, the products of our culture are so rich and so varied that for the first time in human history, you can consume at will, with no external limits.

Consider some facts. According to the U.S. Department of Agriculture people now eat 350 more calories per day than they did just 15 years ago. The average American eats 197 pounds of red meat, poultry and fish per year. Fifty years ago, Americans ate only 133 pounds per year, 64 pounds less per year than now. As quoted in the *Wall Street Journal*, William Dietz, director of nutrition and physical activity at the Centers for Disease Control and Prevention in Atlanta, reports that "as much as 40 percent of the average family's food budget goes for meals eaten outside the home, often at McDonald's and other fast-food establishments. Some 12,000 new foods—including many snack items—are introduced each year, creating a variety of options that tends to lead to overeating."

Food is everywhere. It is so easy to find food and to eat. You can eat at a fast-food restaurant in minutes. You can buy food when you get gas for your car. You can order food by phone or by computer. Companies such as Homelink.com will bring the food to your home. You do not even have to move from your couch.

The same is true for alcohol. It is everywhere. You can buy alcohol in just about any food store, or you can go to a drive-through liquor store to get alcohol without leaving your car. Now you can buy alcohol from a catalog, to be delivered to your home. Or to make it even easier, you can join the wine-of-the-month club and have wine delivered automatically, every month. Now you can purchase alcohol over the Internet, too, providing the convenience of a liquor store at home. It's no wonder that 25 percent of U.S. adults report high levels of alcohol use, high enough to produce an alcohol problem if the drinking continues unchecked.

This abundance has now extended into the realm of sex. Driven by the profit motive, retailers of all types have now started to make sex abundantly available. You can watch television and view a startling amount of sexual explicitness on the networks every night. You can, if you choose, engage in sexually oriented discussions on the Internet or over the telephone. It is possible, using "Web cam" digital technology, to witness live sex acts on the Web. You can use the Internet to find a sex partner, quickly, efficiently, geared to your own preference. In fact, the *Journal of the American Medical Association* reported an outbreak of venereal disease directly traceable to online sex. Sex is becoming as readily available, and as varied, as food.

In one way, this is all a marvelous gift. Freedom from hunger. Freedom from empty hours and loneliness. Freedom from the crushing demands of subsistence living. Now it is up to us to learn how to live with this abundance, in a balanced and healthy way. It is truly possible, if you learn your body and your mind's own natural rules.

Why Do We Consume So Much?

There is a simple answer to the question of why we consume so much. From millions of years of scarcity a powerful message was coded into our human nervous system. That message is: Consume now, because you may not have another opportunity to do so for a while. This is a message of survival. Our ancestors obeyed this message, or else they would not survive. In the world of our ancestors, for millions of years of subsistence living, it was not possible to know when you would next have a meal. You could not tell if your mate would live out the year. You might have to hunt so long and hard that any experience of pleasure and relaxation might only come unpredictably, and at long intervals. Now that message, hard-wired into our brains, is irrelevant at best, damaging and destabilizing at worst.

To make sure that we human beings survived, our nervous system was created to take delight in consumption. It makes sense, really. Our brains are wired in such a way that we automatically experience eating, drinking and having sex as satisfying, appealing and stimulating. These activities are *interesting* to us in the most profound way. The deep, biologic interest, the appetite for food, drink and sex that is a natural part of brain function, protects us from scarcity. The human brain is energized by hunger; it stimulates us to consume to be sure that we have enough, to be sure that we can make it through the inevitable long periods of scarcity until our great efforts next bear fruit.

Appetite for food, sex and drink is deeply wired into your brain. So deeply, that satisfying these appetites is instinctive. Because these brain systems developed in times of scarcity, because consuming was the survival-based, sensible thing to do, there is no instinct to stop. There is no neurological system that was created to instinctively tell you to abstain. There was no need. Resources were so scarce for our ancestors that life forced you to stop eating, to stop drinking and to stop procreating. Our ancestors simply ran out of food, or your mate died, or you had to work so hard to find food that there was no time to drink.

In the world of our ancestors, hundreds of thousands of years ago, you consumed as long as you could, until you ran out of supplies, or until some act of nature forced your hand. Then your brain didn't tell you to stop. Instead, it would tell you to start looking for your next meal, or for a new mate.

The natural rhythm of your brain is to consume as long as you can, until you run out of supplies. Then it is time to plan your next moves. To plan a sequence of activity that will lead to finding food. The rhythm of appetites and abstinence for our ancestors, and now the rhythm within our own brains, is to consume as long as you can and then to plan and work to find more. In balance, your appetites work in harmony with planning and the necessary action of providing the next opportunity to consume. The energy of your appetites, coming from the lower centers of your brain, is linked in balance by the higher centers of your brain, to thinking, to planning and to memory. The result is energized, purposeful planning and action. That is how our ancestors survived. That is how our brains work.

From this fundamental rhythm, it is possible to achieve balance. You can take the energy generated by your appetites and, using it as our ancestors did, channel the energy of your appetites into creative thought, problem solving and taking action. When you understand this brain system in the right way, you can create some rules to follow that will make this happen. There is a logic to this biologic system—if you are open to it.

Eating Helps Her Cope

Debbie consulted with me because she was unhappy and uncomfortable.

"Things have gotten out of hand," she said in her understated way. "It's so many things at once. The kids, my husband, Larry, my home, so many things. You know my parents are sick, too. There is no one to take care of them, so I've taken that on, too. Another responsibility. I just worry and feel bad, especially at night."

"How do you manage?" I asked.

"I just do," Debbie replied. She looked uneasy. "Sometimes it's sort of frantic. I shut it all off at night. I watch TV and I

eat until I fall asleep on the couch. Then the next day I start over again."

Her children, aged eight, ten and twelve, had been the focus of her life. Debbie spent her days driving the kids to school, to soccer, to see friends, to doctors' appointments. Then, when her parents became ill, she would start and end her day at their home, making sure they had food, that they took their medicine and that they were safe for another day. Her parents lived alone in the house that they had spent their lives in, but now could not manage.

Years ago, before the kids were born, Debbie had done assembly work, making computer chips. It had started then. Wound up after her shift at work, she and Larry would relax at home with a bottle of wine and a good dinner. After dinner, they would collapse on the couch, eating cookies, to watch their favorite shows.

"I just got so busy," Debbie explained when I had asked her what had happened to her marriage. She took care of the home, the kids and then her parents. Larry worked hard, as much overtime as he could get, since money was tight. To relax, Larry went hunting on weekends.

"He was never home. I got real lonesome," Debbie told me. "So every night, I had my two glasses of wine. And, like I did when Larry was home with me, I watched TV and ate."

After she had her children, her weight problem worsened.

"I was eating all the time. In the car, while I waited for the kids at the gym, when we went to McDonald's, at night, after the kids were in bed," she told me. Debbie's life had become so frantic and busy, that food was the only source of comfort left to her.

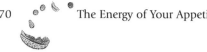
"I sure did love the cakes that Larry would bring home," she told me. "It helped me to feel like he still loved me."

Eating and drinking had become automatic. Despite her obvious weight gain, Debbie did not really notice or think about what she was consuming. Food was a comfort. It was soothing. It had become an expression of affection from her husband. Since Debbie was the sort of person who was sensitive, easily bothered by day-to-day disruptions, food became her solution.

"I want to do something about this. I don't feel right," she told me. As we talked, it became clear that Debbie did not really understand her body and its physical needs. I referred her to a nutritionist. Some education and a diet log helped her see how much she was overeating. But she still didn't lose weight.

"I can see the problem," she told me, "but I still don't know what to do." We talked about the main forces in her life: her kids, her husband and her parents. She discovered that caring for the people she loved set her into a cycle of emotions that led to eating. With her children, it was a mother's worry, with her husband it was loneliness, and when she took care of her parents, she felt sad. Since she was always near food, she would eat. The eating helped her feel better.

Once she understood the way that eating and drinking was prompted by certain feelings and by certain situations, then she could begin to make adjustments. Debbie was a planner by nature. That was, in part, why she worried. Debbie automatically planned. We turned her planning ability on to herself. First, she developed a diet plan that worked. She simplified what she would eat and where she would eat. No more fast food in the car. Instead of thinking about eating when she was in her trigger situations, she would think about calories, meals and the structure of eating. Bringing her planning ability to bear on her appetites helped her cut back. Instead of eating on the run, Debbie would make entries in a diary. She wrote about the situation, what she felt like eating and what she did instead of eating. As she wrote, Debbie developed ways that she could spend more time on projects she enjoyed, such as driving routes and itineraries to shorten the trips with her kids, ideas for helping her parents in their struggle to stay well and to stay in their home. She certainly didn't do everything that she wrote about, but she did some of it. And when she did, it felt good to her, like she was making an impact.

Next, we developed a plan to help her feel rewarded some way other than eating. Debbie was a saver, so the idea she had was to take a big empty jar and every time she thought about food and did not eat, she would reward herself by putting the money she would have spent on food into the jar. When she had saved enough, Debbie would treat herself to some new clothes.

As she gained confidence in herself, as she no longer was assuaged by food, Debbie discovered how lonely she was, and how upset she was that Larry was not more helpful with her parents. Although Larry was a good husband and provider, he was not home enough, and he did not help her enough. She started to talk with Larry. Over time, and with the help of some couples counseling, Larry responded.

"I'm getting there," Debbie told me. Indeed she was. She had lost fifty pounds, and she had a renewed enthusiasm for her life. She was putting her life back into balance.

What worked for Debbie? How did she use her mind to balance her appetites? She did so by using her natural rules.

Debbie's Rules for the Energy of Her Appetites

1. *Simplify what she eats and where she eats.*
2. *Recognize her eating triggers—feeling worried, lonely or sad.*
3. *Make plans to solve problems instead of eating.*
4. *Reward herself with money and clothes.*
5. *Don't accept food as a substitute for a real relationship. Ask her husband for what she really needs.*

These are natural rules that balanced her automatic instincts to consume. That is how Debbie restored a natural balance in her life, the natural balance that comes from a harmonious rhythm of excitation and inhibition, different parts of your brain and your mind working together in a fluid harmony and in balance. Using her rules, Debbie was able to structure and channel the energy of her appetites. She was able to balance her appetites by shifting her energy away from eating and drinking; shifting the energy of her appetites toward constructive action that made sense in her life.

Let's look a little further, to understand the basis for Debbie's rules of appetite balance.

Appetites, Energy and Balance

Your body is poised to be hungry. Your cells cry out for food. It is a condition of living. In the center of your brain, the nerve cells that create your appetites stand on guard and ready for any sign of need. When these nerve cells sense the slightest change in the hunger signals from your body, then your appetite is activated. Your brain and your mind become energized by your hunger.

The same is true for sex. The very same cells in the center of your brain continuously watch for signals from your body that indicate that you are ready to procreate, to take the necessary steps to reproduce life. The signals are hormonal. When your appetite center senses the right hormones, it stimulates your appetite for sex.

And even though drinking alcohol is not essential to life, through some quirk of nature, the need to drink alcohol, the appetite to drink, is in the same part of the brain. It works the same way.

Your appetite for food, for drink and for sex are, for the most part, interchangeable. Forty percent of people with a sexual problem will also have a problem with alcohol. Thirty-eight percent will also have a problem with food. Twenty-five percent of women with eating problems will also have a problem with alcohol.

Listen to the words of Caroline Knapp, describing the problem in her book, *Drinking: A Love Story.*

> You hear about women who became bulimic or anorexic in high school, then established some kind of equilibrium around food when or after they

started drinking. For men it's usually other drugs, most often pot or cocaine, or it's gambling. Sometimes it's a more obscure behavior.

The facts are that people who have a balance problem with one type of appetite also tend to have problems with the others. From the standpoint of the way that your brain works, all three types of appetites are generated and controlled in the same way.

The message from your appetite center is as simple as it is continuous. Your appetite centers were created by nature to tell your body and your mind to eat when you can, to have sex when you can, to drink when you can. When your appetite center senses hunger, it activates and energizes the higher centers of your brain, not just to consume but to take action. That is how appetites are balanced: The energy of your hunger is balanced by taking action. In the language of your brain, abstinence is really all about planning, problem solving and taking action.

Of course, like everything in your body and in your mind, it is not quite that simple. Because survival is so important, the strength and persistence of your appetite can change. While there is not much need for a variation in your appetites now, for our ancestors, appetites varied in harmony with changes in the environment, with changes in the circumstances of life. Over tens of thousands of years, our brains developed so that appetite levels were exquisitely responsive to the need to survive. Now we live with the accumulated biologic experience of our ancestors. This means that the strength and persistence of your appetites can vary over a wide range, depending on a number of factors.

All of this helped our ancestors to survive. For us, since survival is not at issue, these biologic determinants of appetite guarantee that we will have trouble living in balance. Abundance, in the way that we experience it today, does not satisfy our appetites. In the biology of your brain, consumption does not decrease your appetite. In some ways, the opposite is true. Certain kinds of abundance can actually increase the strength of your appetites. And in our culture, abundance is everywhere: from the fast-food restaurants on every corner, to the thousands of images of beautiful, sexually desirable men and women we see in the media every day, to the ease and convenience of locating a drink.

The factors that strengthen your appetites are listed on the chart below.

Factors That Increase Appetite

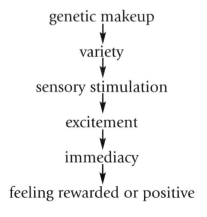

genetic makeup
↓
variety
↓
sensory stimulation
↓
excitement
↓
immediacy
↓
feeling rewarded or positive

The good news is that you can use the factors that affect the strength of your appetite to create some natural rules to guide you to a healthy balance. Let's discuss each of these factors in turn.

Genetics

The strength of your appetite for food, sex and drink is an inherited characteristic, much like your need for sleep. Your level of appetite is unique to you, programmed by your genes, responding to some environmental factor that was present in the life of your ancestors, eons ago. For example, if your ancestors lived in a far northern climate, then a strong appetite would have helped them consume enough to live through long stretches of snowy, cold weather. Cold weather living burns many more calories per day than living in a warm climate. If you now live in a warm climate, the intense level of your appetites may not fit your circumstance.

If you are blessed with strong appetites, in today's world of abundance you can easily fall out of balance through overconsuming. Answer the following questions to gauge how strong your appetites are.

How Strong Are Your Appetites?

1. Do you struggle with feeling hungry much of the time?	yes	no
2. Are you overweight?	yes	no
3. Do you look forward to eating, or do you think about food much of the day?	yes	no
4. Once you start eating, do you have trouble stopping?	yes	no
5. Are most of your family members overweight?	yes	no
6. Do you feel driven to engage in sexual activity?	yes	no
7. Do you find yourself thinking about sexual activity much of the day?	yes	no
8. Does engaging in or thinking about sexual activity interfere with other parts of your life?	yes	no
9. Do find yourself often thinking about having a drink?	yes	no
10. Do you drink every day?	yes	no
11. Does alcohol cause problems in your life?	yes	no
12. Once you start drinking, do you have trouble stopping?	yes	no

---

If you answered yes to three or more of these questions, then, in all likelihood, you have strong appetites. You inherited strong appetites from your ancestors. In a way, this can be a good thing. Strong appetites are like a life force from within. You hunger for life and all that it brings. Your body and your mind were created with powerful urges; the real purpose of these urges, of your appetites, is to energize you to seek life-sustaining resources and to enrich life.

What can you do about this? Plenty—once you fully

understand how biologically strong your appetites are. First of all, you can give yourself a break. You may be prone to gaining weight, or to drinking or to having affairs because of your biology—not because you are a bad person. Having strong appetites is like being left-handed. It is just the way you are made. The trick is to learn to adjust. Educate yourself; use your mind to fully understand how strong your appetites are; learn to consume what you need and not what you want; learn to shift the energy of your appetites onto creative, purposeful, enriching activity, activity that may not have anything to do with eating, drinking or having sex.

This leads to the first rule:

Rule #1: Consume Only What You Need and Not What You Want

Follow this rule by educating yourself. That will help your thinking brain to modulate and control the energy of your appetites from the lower centers of your brain.

Calculate how much food you really need. Try to live with a moderate amount of alcohol use. This is generally thought to be the equivalent of six glasses of wine per week. Engage in sexual activity only to the degree that it does not interfere with your life, your health or your partner's happiness.

This approach sounds simple-minded because it is. Once you understand that much of your consumption is unnecessary, driven only by the biologic power of your appetites, then it becomes easier to balance. How? By learning to redirect the energy of your appetites. That is the subject of the rest of this chapter. The remaining sections, the remaining rules of living, are all about how to use your mind to turn the power and passion of your appetites away from consumption and toward a healthy balance in your life.

Variety

A variety of experience stimulates your appetites. You can see this whenever you have a multicourse meal. Each time the table is cleared and a new food or wine is served, you feel a renewed appetite. The same is true for sexual encounters. You can see this in our intense attraction to sexually oriented content in the media.

Why? It is because variety, in some settings, helps survival. Different foods provide different nutrients. Having different sexual partners increases the likelihood of procreation especially if the death rate of reproduction is high (as it was until one hundred years ago). Variety is not important for survival now. You can get all the nutrients you need by taking vitamins and eating Power Bars. Nutritional survival does not require variety. With the advent of modern medicine, the likelihood that your spouse or your children will die within the year is remote. There is no need to try and reproduce at all costs. Since the appetite for drinking uses the same appetite structures in the brain, while drinking alcohol has no survival value, your appetite for drinking increases with variety.

Rule #2: Simplify What You Consume

Give yourself fewer choices to make it easier to abstain. To help your appetite to subside naturally, to make it easier to shift your attention away from food, sex or drink on to productive activity, a natural step to take is to simplify what you consume. Decrease the variety of what you consume and your appetite will naturally decrease.

Sensory Stimulation

Sensory interest—sight, sounds, touch or pleasant fragrance—can stimulate your appetite. Think of the wine connoisseur who reacts to the color and fragrance of wine in addition to the varied tastes of the wine on his or her palate. The same is true for food. Expert chefs know that the "presentation" of food, the way it looks, can be as important as the way it tastes. Sensory stimulation had the same survival value to our ancestors as variety. Interesting sights, sounds, smells and touch, by stimulating appetite, helped our ancestors consume with sufficient quantity and variety to ensure that they survived.

Retailers and advertisers know this natural law. We are bombarded by sensually stimulating images of food, sex and drink all day long. To attract us to buy, to consume, the sensual pleasures of our abundant world are enhanced. They are used to create an appetite for consumption. And it works. Just think of how often you may have been motivated to eat as a result of seeing an advertisement on television. Or how many times have you bought more food than you wanted at a store, because it looked so good and smelled so delicious.

But if you subtract the sensory input, your appetite can wane. If you make the subject of your appetite less interesting, then you will be more easily satisfied.

Rule #3: Focus on Your Needs and Not Solely on Your Senses

With alcohol, the way you simplify is to avoid drinking. Over time, your senses will take delight in other things. When you do not drink, you will find that you have energy and interest for a world of activity. With eating, the trick is to eat simpler foods when you want to control your intake. To cut down on unnecessary eating, follow a diet plan that limits your exposure to foods that delight and overload your senses. By all means eat these pleasurable foods, but do so as part of a total diet plan.

Excitement

When you begin to associate eating, drinking or having sex with excitement, it can enhance your appetite. For some, the "thrill of the chase" is the most compelling part of satisfying an appetite. This is most evident with sexual appetites. It is commonly a part of drinking too much; the act of drinking becomes strongly associated with the fun of socializing or being at a party. This is a matter of training or learning. If you learn to associate eating or drinking with a type of excitement, then after a time, the eating or drinking itself begins to create some of the excitement. The good news is that you can train yourself to undo this

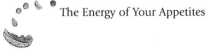
association. Learning to detach the appetite from the source of the excitement can help make your appetite more controllable. It also will help you find excitement elsewhere in your life. When you free up the energy that comes from hunger, you will find it easier to think creatively, to find excitement in other parts of your life.

In our consumption-oriented society, much of the excitement in life has been linked to eating, drinking or having sex. Having hot dogs is as much a part of the ball-game as the baseball game itself. Sexual content in music and movies is now the norm. And we expect to drink any time we are having fun. Liquor is inextricably tied to every form of entertainment and pleasure. For us, consumption is excitement.

Rule #4: Separate Excitement from Consumption

Find other activities or aspects of activities that are exciting to you. Try to enjoy movies and video for the plot and the music, not for the sex. When you go to a ball-game, enjoy the athletic competition and not the hot dog. Better yet, try to develop some excitement in ways that are completely separate from eating, drinking and having sex . . . like rock climbing or singing in a choir or the excitement of creating something new.

Immediacy

Immediacy, or being surrounded by the object of your appetite, can make your desire skyrocket. But having to wait tends to dull your desire. After a time, it just does not seem worth it. Remember, your appetite tells you to consume if you can, so if you are surrounded by food, or by drink, or by sex, expect that your appetite will be harder to balance.

Conversely, if you structure your exposure to food, drink and sex, then you can balance your appetites more easily.

Rule #5: Balance Your Appetites by Structuring When You Consume and How You Consume

You may want to avoid eating in your car or in front of the TV. You could limit the length of time you eat, or limit the times of day that you eat. If sex is a problem, you might only watch sexually oriented videos with your spouse. Or you could avoid sexually oriented chat rooms on the Internet. The trick to applying this rule is to provide yourself with times and places that are free of consumption.

Feeling Rewarded

The last factor may be the strongest factor for we humans. It is certainly a uniquely human factor. That is the psychologic value of whatever it is you are hungry for. Think about how much hungrier you feel at the prospect of a gourmet meal at a well-known four-star restaurant. Think about how your sex drive gets increased at the thought of a famous and impossibly attractive movie star. In more everyday terms, think about how you are more likely to eat, to drink or to have sex if it feels like a treat or a reward. When this happens, it is because the higher centers of your brain and mind are chiming in, telling you to "do this because it is really important." Your brain believes that consumption that feels rewarding or important is good for your survival; consequently, your appetites increase.

This response is also a matter of learning. Just as you can learn to be rewarded by certain foods, you can unlearn this response. You can train yourself to be rewarded in a healthier way, so that it becomes easier to balance your appetite with the right amount of abstinence.

The next rule of balanced appetites comes from this connection.

Rule #6: Unlink Eating, Drinking and Having Sex from Any Sense of Reward

Find other activities that are rewarding, and use them to avoid consuming. Debbie found a way to reward herself with money and clothes. You could just as well reward yourself with a phone call to a friend. You could reward yourself with concert tickets. You could reward yourself by finding time to play with your kids. You could reward yourself by finally going back to school. By using your mind, you can discover a world of interest and activity that is rewarding to you. Then you can successfully replace appetite-driven consumption with the satisfaction that comes from accomplishment.

Thinking Balances Appetites

It is so easy to consume. You can find food, drink or sexual activity (at least in the media) in minutes, no matter what time of day it is, or where you are. With your appetites whetted by the proximity, the sensory stimulation and the excitement of our consumer culture, the natural thing to do is to eat, to drink or to engage in sexual activity.

That is too bad. A world of experience is being camouflaged by hunger. A lifetime of thought, emotional reaction and human creativity is being dulled by satiation. Whatever you are feeling, whatever experience may be stimulating your thoughts, whatever plans you may be hatching, you may never take action because it is so easy to consume. Why? It is because the natural response to hunger, the natural response to a stimulated appetite, is to plan, to think, to dream and to take action—not to consume. When your appetite is stimulated, it triggers the higher centers in your brain to start working, to think about creative ways to handle your hunger. When you consume, you short-circuit this process; when you satisfy an appetite, you are simply responding to a demand from the older, instinctive parts of your brain. And by satisfying your appetite, you have stopped the natural process of creative planning and problem solving. You will have drained the energy away from your thinking brain. You will have unlinked appetite and energy from thinking.

The natural balance of appetites is actually like this:

1. Hunger leads to creative planning.
2. Planning leads to taking action.
3. Taking action leads to finding food, drink and a mate.
4. Once you have found what you need, then you consume.

In modern life, the short-circuited pathway of unlimited consumption looks like this:

1. Hunger leads directly to consumption.

There is just so much to do. As you push hard, following your passion, living in today's fast-paced, demanding world, it leaves you out of balance. If there is one thing that our culture excels at, one thing that truly sets our culture apart, it is that in our culture and our society, we are each provided with the opportunity to consume to our heart's content. And that is what causes us to have trouble with the balance of appetites.

No matter what your situation, no matter what is troubling you or turning you on, there is always a ready fix—to eat, to drink or to engage in sexually oriented activity. Sometimes the proximity of food, drink and sex will keep you from taking action; it short-circuits the natural planning response. Sometimes it will not; even though you are distracted toward consumption, you still find a way to take action. But what is clear is that the ready availability of food, drink and sex unbalances your appetite. It causes you to live with unhealthy patterns of consumption.

Why? Because it feels good. At the deepest levels of your nervous system, eating, drinking and having sex activates a pleasure response. That is your brain's way of saying, "Everything is okay. I'll live another day." Regardless of what is unsettling to you, consuming makes you feel better. At least for a while. Because it is so easy to consume, you can lose your balance and become stuck in a cycle of consuming, camouflaging the fact that you don't feel right.

But the problem leads to a natural solution. Just as satisfying your appetite can block you from understanding your problems and taking action, understanding your problems and taking action can balance your appetite. In the way that your brain is made, the energy of your appetites, from the older parts of your brain, is balanced by thought, planning and action. That is the secret of balancing your appetites. You can diminish and control your appetites somewhat, using the natural rules I've outlined above. *But to truly balance your appetites, you must use your mind . . . to think, to plan and to take action instead of consuming.* When you do, you will find that you are much more likely to live with a pattern of balanced consumption. It was true for our ancestors. They had no choice. Subsistence living forced them into balance. For our ancestors, hunger was balanced by planning, creative problem solving and taking action, so that they could find food and a mate. Using these natural rules of balance, it can be true for you.

The last rule for balancing the energy of your mind, for a healthy balance of appetites and abstinence, comes directly from the way that your brain was created to work.

It was created to use the energy from your older, instinctive brain, in balance with the higher centers of your brain, in balance with your ability to think, to plan and take action. Here is the rule.

Rule #7: Balance the Energy of Your Appetites by Using Your Mind; Think, Plan and Take Action Instead of Consuming

You can put this rule into effect by combining it with the rules you have learned from earlier chapters. Take the energy of your appetites and combine it with what you know about being with people, about movement and about using your tools. Make the structure of your mind in balance; use your own unique style, preferences and abilities; use the rules of your own natural balance to channel the energy of your appetites into a creative force. Use your mind to think, to plan and to take action in the way that is right for you and, by doing so, use the energy of your appetites in a healthy balance. After all, that is how your brain was created to function.

Listen to Jim's story. You will see how Jim reestablished balance in his life by using this natural rule.

Using Alcohol to Escape

He did not look well when he first came to see me. There was a bloated, puffiness around Jim's eyes. His skin was sallow and flecked with the telltale red marks of burst blood vessels. Jim consulted me because he felt depressed. Stuck in a demanding job that was beneath his abilities, Jim worked long hours to make his numbers, often as much as twelve to fourteen hours per day. By the time he got home, he was alone; his kids were in bed, his wife Barbara was engrossed in her sewing. He had fallen into a pattern of drinking beer, eating take-out pizza and watching grade-B movies on cable TV.

"At the end of the day, I feel so wired that beer and pizza is what I need to relax," he told me. "If I could just get a new job, things would be better."

Barbara asked him to spend more time at home. She asked him to cut back on the beer he was drinking. Jim tried. But it didn't work. He began to stop at O'Connor's Pub on the way home, to have a few beers to calm down after work. He didn't get home any earlier, but at least he felt better by the time he got home.

He thought it was all due to work. But as we dug deeper, a different picture emerged. About five years before, Jim's older brother had died suddenly. A car accident had taken his life. Steve had been like a father to Jim; ten years older than Jim, Steve had stepped in to help when their mom had divorced their dad. Jim's dad had been an alcoholic. A man of violent temper, he had paralyzed the home with fear. He died two years after the divorce, in a car accident, while drunk; this caused Jim to have a confusing mix of feelings: sadness, for sure, relief, a strange sense of guilt.

Steve's sudden death hit Jim with a terrible force. After the funeral, Jim focused intensely on work. Driven by a powerful ambition to produce, the long hours began. During lunchtime meetings, over a beer or two, he found himself attracted to Sally, a member of his team. Sally was just a few years out of college; she was beautiful, flush with the energy and vigor of being young, unattached and confident. She and Jim had an affair.

When his boss found out, Jim decided that it was time to stop. He and Sally agreed it was for the best. Instead, Jim worked harder, and his drinking increased. Barbara never knew. Jim started to avoid her; he felt so badly. Having an extramarital affair was something he could not condone; there was no way for him to understand what happened, nor to talk about it with Barbara. He spent more time alone, drinking beer, in front of the TV. His life was out of balance.

To start Jim on the road to recovery, we set up some rules designed to limit his drinking. Jim's appetite for drinking was constantly stimulated by the facts of his day-to-day life. To start balancing the energy of his appetite, and to begin the process of channeling this energy toward planning and taking action, we used appetite rules one through six, tailoring the rules to fit his life.

Jim's Rules for Managing Drinking

1. *Limit his drinking to six beers per week. This was a healthy amount for Jim. More than six beers led to drinking too much. Stopping all beer entirely seemed like an impossible sacrifice. So we settled on six.*
2. *Drink only light beer. Jim knew that the taste of light beer would limit the amount he drank, because after he had two, he didn't want any more. This rule worked by decreasing the sensory pleasure of drinking.*
3. *Drink only in restaurants and only with Carol. This rule helped Jim by controlling when and where he drank. It also separated drinking from work, helping him to separate the emotional roller-coaster of work from his experience of drinking alcohol.*
4. *Get a massage after work. Jim knew that drinking had become a reward for a hard day's work. In his mind, it also helped him relax. We came up with a plan. Jim would save the money he would have spent drinking and use it to reward himself with an after-work massage. This felt like a reward for Jim, and it helped him to relax.*

Jim worked these rules for a month. They helped, but not enough. He had been able to cut back, but every day was a battle against the craving for alcohol.

"It's wearing me out, Doc," Jim told me. "I'm thinking about when I can have a few beers, all day long."

We talked about what had happened at the same time as he started to have trouble. We talked about his brother, Steve, about Carol and about work. Jim thought there might be a connection. I proposed another rule of balance. Since Jim worked in computers, he always had a laptop with him. This was the tool we chose to use. I had Jim create three files, labeled Steve, Carol and work. Then whenever he felt a craving for alcohol, he was to open these files and write down the thoughts that came to him in these matters.

It was not easy. As Jim wrote, his cravings subsided—but he felt pain instead. There was sadness and a sense of feeling all alone in his world linked to Steve's death. There was intense guilt about deceiving Carol, and about not being there for his kids. There was anger and dissatisfaction about the ill treatment he had received at work.

But from these feelings came ideas and plans. Recalling how Steve had supported him when he had been on a swim team and how good that felt, Jim decide to volunteer to coach the swim team at the YMCA and to get his own kids involved. He knew that he had a lot to make up to Carol. He talked with Carol, trying his best to explain everything. Understandably, she was hurt and angry but after talking with her friends, Carol began to forgive Jim. To rekindle their relationship they planned a trip for the two of them to the south of France, a place that Carol loved. He wrote a new résumé, outlining all that he had accomplished at work. Then he sent it off, looking for a better job.

Jim used the energy that came from his hunger for alcohol to creatively think about his problems. As he did, it became easier to abstain. It became easier to follow the other rules of appetite balance that we had created for him.

To truly balance your appetites, you must use your mind to think, to plan and to take action instead of consuming.

That is how your brain works. A natural balance of the stimulation of your appetites, channeled into useful thought, planning and action. That is how Jim rebalanced his life. He used his mind to balance the power of his appetites.

Here are the rules for balancing the energy of your appetites with the power and creativity of your mind.

The Energy of Your Appetites Self-Test

Take this test to see if you are out of balance. If you answer yes to two or more questions, then you may have a problem with appetite balance. To improve your balance, try to incorporate the rules in this chapter as well as the tips to follow.

1. Do you eat, drink alcohol or engage in sex, at times simply by habit, even when you don't have a physical need?   yes   no
2. Have you been unsuccessful in trying to cut down on the amount that you eat, drink or have sex?   yes   no
3. Do you feel that eating, drinking or having sex is a significant source of excitement and reward for you?   yes   no

4. Do you often find it hard to control
   your appetites because you are surrounded
   by food, by alcohol or by sexually
   oriented materials?   yes   no

Tips to Balance the Energy
of Your Appetites

Here is a list of tips to help you to balance the energy generated by your appetites and, using this natural energy source
as our ancestors did, channel the energy of your appetites
into creative thought, problem solving and taking action.

Try some of these tips in the fourth week of your balance program. It is not necessary to go on a diet, or to
abstain from activities that give you pleasure. Instead you
can use these tips to help yourself begin to find a healthy
balance; gain a better understanding of how much you
may eat, drink and have sex—and how much you should
abstain. Learn to creatively use your natural energy,
instead of consuming.

1. Keep a chart of how you are consuming. This
   simple tool is one of the most effective ways to
   redirect strong appetites and reduce your consumption, whether it is an appetite for food, drink
   or sex. Charting your consumption will work, even
   if you are unable to do anything else! Keep it
   simple to make it work. Your chart can be as

simple as a small spiral notepad that you can buy for under a dollar. Then list what you consume and when. By doing this, you are using a powerful, thought-based tool, to bring your patterns of consumption under conscious control.

2. Set aside time for sex. Whether you struggle with too much sexual activity or too little, planning your sexual activity can have a powerful effect on your appetite. Make it fun, add whatever safe sensory pleasure you like. By doing so, you structure the way you satisfy this basic appetite.

4. Do not drink more than one piña colada, fruit daiquiri, sombrero, tequila sunrise or any other sweet alcoholic drink at a sitting. Why? Because the sugary flavor, the color and the fun of these drinks can cause you to drink more alcohol than you may want. If you are at a social function where you would like to drink, then drink alcohol in a form that does not taste that good.

5. Enjoy beauty, wherever you may find it. Take in the sensual pleasures that are freely available in our beautiful world: the beauty of nature, the beauty of the creative arts, the beauty of fashion, the beauty of architecture, the beauty of children at play. You can redirect the energy of your appetites by developing an aesthetic sense, an appreciation of what you find to be beautiful in your world. When you do so, you are truly satisfying your appetites, but you are doing so in a way that is in balance with

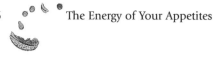

your higher brain functions. An appreciation of beauty is one of the gifts of being human.

6. Write down a problem that you want to solve, along with the tools you might use to solve it. Keep this reminder handy. When you feel your appetite increasing, use the energy of the appetite to develop creative solutions to your problem. Simple, concrete, day-to-day problems work best. For example, one problem might be how to influence your child to spend less time playing with his/her Game Boy. If one of your tools is that you enjoy reading, as a form of relaxation, then perhaps you might find a fun and interesting story to read to your child. Then when you feel your appetite rising, you could go to a bookstore, or get on the Internet to look for just the right book to read to your child.

7. Eat frequent small, nutritious meals. Scientists have proven that this pattern of eating is the healthiest. It also takes advantage of your natural rules by providing you with food in a way that does not stimulate you to excess eating. "Grazing" has gotten a bad name in the popular press, because of the association with fast foods and unhealthy foods. But if you consume frequent small meals, like a piece of fruit and some crackers, or a Power Bar and a juice drink, you may actually eat less, feel healthier and lose weight. One caution, when you eat in this pattern you replace your three meals a day with the frequent small meals. It

will not work if you eat frequent small meals and your regular three meals per day.

8. Drink water. Water, of course, is calorie free, totally healthy, and available everywhere. It is the ideal substance to consume on the run. When you drink a tall, cool glass of water, the act of drinking, the fullness of the water in your stomach, and the way that water quenches your thirst will diminish your appetite for food, drink and even for sex (although water in the form of a cold shower may work best for sex).

9. Play board games or card games with your family or your friends. The intellectual challenge of a good game, the pleasure of spending time with people you care about in a fun activity and the pleasures of competition make this type of activity a natural and balanced reward for the energy of your appetites. But remember, when you are playing, leave the potato chips, the beer and the peanuts in the closet. In the evenings, instead of sitting on the couch with a beer, or glass of wine and a bag of chips, gather your friends or family for a lively game that you all can enjoy.

10. Count your money. When an appetite strikes, try counting your money. Balance your checkbook, finally roll those pennies, call your bank for your balances, figure out how much you spend on everything. Why? Because money is rewarding. It may be one of the only things that is more of a motivator, for many people, than food, alcohol

and sex. Counting your money can calm your nerves by telling you where you really stand. But what if counting your money makes you nervous because of how tight your finances are? Then you will have real focus for using the energy of your appetites in creative problem solving. If money is tight, then get "money hungry" and, instead of eating, drinking or having sex, figure how to improve your finances.

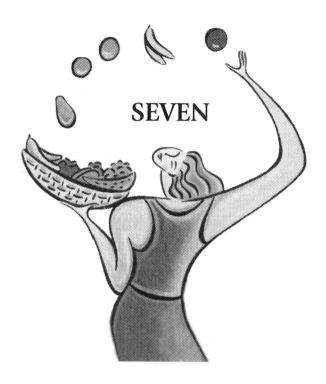

SEVEN

System 5:
Thinking and Feeling

Certain aspects of the process of emotion and feelings are indispensable for rationality. At their best feelings point us in the proper direction, take us to the appropriate place in a decision-making space, where we may put the instruments of logic to good use.

Antonio R. Damasio, *Descartés Error*

Emotion Is the Energy of Thought

What turns you on? Do you greet each day with enthusiasm and interest? Do you have a clear sense of what to do? Is your life enjoyable? Are the events of your day meaningful and rewarding? Or does life seem dull, routine and uninteresting? Do you have trouble deciding what to do or how to start? Is the emotion missing from your day, appearing only when you become angered, irritable or worried by the next deadline, by traffic, by overcrowded airplanes or by the million little demands that life places before you?

These are questions of balance; a flowing, rhythmic and harmonious balance. You see, your brain was created to work that way. Feeling and thought. Your thinking powered by emotion; emotion guided by your intellect. It can flow in both directions.

Here are some facts to guide us.

- Educational specialist Priscilla Vail, in her book *Emotion: The On/Off Switch for Learning,* describes the way in which emotion, excitement, interest and enthusiasm improve learning. She describes an effective system for teaching children, by combining emotional involvement with standard school subjects. Educators now understand the key role of emotion to improve learning.
- Psychiatrist Edward Hallowell, M.D., has studied factors that improve school performance in teenagers. His findings: Emotional attachment, a quality that

he calls connectedness, to family, to school and to friends, is the best predictor of superior school performance.

- The research of neurologist Antonio Damasio, M.D., has proven that body and mind function as a single unit. He calls his theory the somatic marker hypothesis which says that physical sensation and emotional reactions provide the framework on which rational thought and logic is built.
- Powerful brain imaging machines like the PET scanner show that when your mind is active with an interesting or enjoyable mental task, the brain areas for rational thought and the brain areas for emotion and pleasure light up together, proving that they function as a single circuit.

So you can see that a feeling or emotion combines a physical sensation and a thought that gives it meaning. You need both. Different emotions are created by your physical reactions in the context and meaning of different situations in your life.

These physical reactions are lightning fast. Your brain takes in all the sensation that it can and translates it instantly into a physical reaction. This reaction becomes a feeling when you think about what has just happened. For example, if your heart is racing, your muscles tense, your stomach is doing flip-flops and you are on a roller coaster at Six Flags, then you interpret this as fun.

Now take the same physical sensations in your boss's office and you are likely to interpret this same physical reaction as fear. Once your brain or your intellect figures out what is going on, then you develop a plan of action. If you are on the roller coaster, you hold on tight and laugh. But if you are in your boss's office, you start to develop a plan to solve the problem: Should you explain? Should you make a pitch? Should you prepare a résumé because you are about to be fired?

The physical sensations happen automatically. Your senses collect information and send it to lower centers in your brain, in the brain stem. These same brain centers then produce a physical reaction.

At the same time, the message is relayed to higher centers in your brain, in your neocortex, where the message is interpreted. Meaning is applied. You think about your situation and how you are feeling. The stronger the physical reaction, the more powerful the feeling. And then the more likely you are to take action, to do something about how you are feeling. Here is a diagram to show how this works.

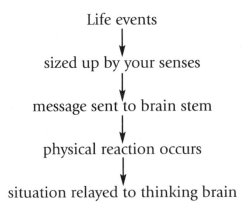

Life events

↓

sized up by your senses

↓

message sent to brain stem

↓

physical reaction occurs

↓

situation relayed to thinking brain

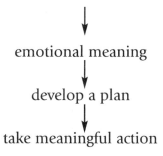

emotional meaning

develop a plan

take meaningful action

This is how emotion and intellect come together. This is how your brain works in balance: thinking powered by feeling; emotion guided and given meaning by thought.

It makes sense when you think about it. In a world of experience and sensation; in a world of possibility, your brain has been created to fluidly respond, to decide what to do, to develop a feeling about what is important and to motivate you to act.

It certainly made sense in the prehistoric world of our ancestors. In those days of subsistence living, correctly interpreting physical reactions was essential to life. Knowing the difference between the excitement of a successful hunt and the fear of being close to a dangerous animal could mean the difference between finding a meal and being turned into a meal. Knowing the difference between the pleasure of making warm clothing and the pleasure of making a meal could mean the difference between having warm clothing when you needed it or being exposed to killing cold. Knowing the difference between the warm bond of love and the blushing discomfort of shame could mean the difference between living in the comfort of a village or being cast out, to fend for yourself as a misfit.

So the human brain developed in this way. Thinking powered by feeling; emotion guided by thought. In balance. And it is there that we shall look for the natural rules for the healthy balance of thinking and feeling. Here is a story about Christopher that will help you to see what I mean.

Divorced and Depressed

"I need help," Christopher told me. "I don't feel much like getting out of bed, except to go to work and to deal with the essentials. You know, getting food, going to the drycleaner and so forth."

Slouched in the chair, his clothes looking as though he had slept in them, mustache drooping over his upper lip, Christopher spoke in a soft monotone voice. He sounded flat.

Divorced for about four years, he lived alone, in an apartment near work. And work he did—over eighty hours per week. Except when he had his daughter with him, which was seldom. He felt awkward with her and a little bored. Whatever interested his ten-year-old daughter was a mystery to him. The problem began when he was married. As Karen and Hannah spent time together, playing with Hannah's Barbie dolls, playing dress-up, going to play dates, Christopher felt more and more isolated. He could not figure out how to fit in at home. He did not find any of it interesting or appealing to him. He became preoccupied by his work, growing distant and angry.

"I guess I'm good at what I do. That's what they tell me. All

I can see is the numbers. At least they make sense to me."

I asked Christopher if there was anything that he got excited about, anything that he enjoyed.

"About the only time I feel anything is when I'm fighting with my ex-wife. She'll call me just about any time to fight. Sometimes I think I ought to just throw my cell phone in the trash. But then she'd probably fight with me by e-mail."

Exact and demanding by nature, Christopher worked tracking inventory for a big chain store. By following the numbers, he balanced the flow of goods, making sure that the supply of clothing from his vendors matched the sales needs for the stores.

"It's all the same, the numbers I mean, it's just data sets. The numbers come to me, I analyze them, push a few buttons and the inventory flows. The work is simple, but it's high volume so there is a lot of pressure to perform. There's a real routine to it."

Christopher was good at his job, but his life had fallen seriously out of balance. Karen, his ex-wife, had pushed for the divorce because of his temper. He would come home from work and erupt at her and at their daughter, Hannah. Over little things, insignificant things, every night the arguments started. I asked him why.

"It's just that things at home didn't make sense. All day long I work on numbers, making sure that everything goes to the right places, then I would get home and nothing is right. The dishes aren't done, the beds aren't made, there's nothing to eat. So I blew up at Karen. Probably too much. Now we're divorced, and still all we do is fight."

With his demanding, aggressive style, Christopher had quickly found success in business. His skills were in demand. And it led him into a career path he did not like. He had *wanted to be a buyer, to find the right clothing for the stores, bargaining hard for a good price. The excitement of the open market. Then to maybe one day open his own store. Instead, he was locked into his job managing inventory. He made too much money to quit. Dulled by the routine, dissatisfied with the work, he gave up on his dream.*

And as the never-ending demands of his job took over, he lost interest in other parts of his life. Everything became a bother. He started to fight with his wife and to yell at his daughter. He had lost his balance. The day-to-day grind of analyzing inventory, the hours he spent working at a task he did not like, the pressures to perform all had taken a toll. His life had become a confusing mix of boredom, apathy and anger.

The path to balance for Christopher began with painting. I had asked him to recall an activity that had given him pleasure. As a student in college, he had taken up landscape painting, to pass the time, to help him to relax, to balance the business courses he was taking. So I asked him to set aside time to paint. Since his evenings were empty, it was easy to find the time. The hard part was that as he painted, he would begin to cry.

"It's been so long since I enjoyed anything. I feel like such a fool," he told me. I encouraged him to persist. He did. And as he painted, the colors, the texture of the paint, the gracefully evolving pictures helped him relax and feel alive.

Although the emotional energy from painting felt painful to Christopher at times, we were able to use some of it to help him in other ways. We talked for a time about what was important to him. Here is what Christopher decided.

What mattered to Christopher:

- improving the relationship with his daughter Hannah
- making money
- stopping the fights with Karen
- finding a source of enjoyment in his life.

The next step for Christopher was to make a plan; he needed to find a way to solve the problem of how to become involved with things that really mattered to him. When he got comfortable with the idea that his job mattered because of the amount of money he made, then possibilities opened up in his mind. He knew that Hannah loved to shop and that she loved dolls. So Christopher decided that he and Hannah could develop a hobby business, buying and selling dolls. He financed it at the start with money he had saved. It didn't take much. Hannah began to come to visit him more often, to pore over trade publications and to look for auctions on the Internet. Christopher found that he had a natural network of connections at work, through relationships with his producers. At work, he began to give himself ten-minute breaks from his inventory control, to e-mail his suppliers about doll auctions and rare finds.

Christopher began to have fun. He looked forward to the time he spent with Hannah. As his enjoyment grew, he became freer with his money, agreeing to extra expenses in discussions with Karen and moving their relationship onto better footing. There was a natural change in his pattern of reactions. Since he energetically pursued deals, since he was aggressively hunting and bargaining for rare and collectible dolls, Christopher found it easier to be patient with the rest of his life. He focused his creative, demanding energies on the marketplace for his rare and collectible dolls.

"I had been so focused on the numbers, that I had lost sight of a few things," he told me. "I had forgotten how much fun it is to try to make a deal. It kind of came back to me the other day. I wanted a job that paid well, so I could use the money to start a business. Maybe buying and selling antiques. But you know how it is, the job sort of took over my life." Sad that he hadn't caught on sooner, Christopher still felt better about his life.

He had lost the balance of feeling and thinking. He had been swept away into a world of calculations that had no meaning, a world of unfeeling routine. Through our discussions, and some trial and error, Christopher learned how to reconnect his passion to his life. He reconnected thinking and feeling.

Starting simply, with painting, he got in touch with a sense of creative pleasure he had lost. Painting gave him a tool to re-engage with his feelings after a day spent with his numbers at work.

Then he developed a plan to use two strong emotions to energize a map for his life. When honest with himself, Christopher was proud of the amount of money he made. It was a source of accomplishment and satisfaction. This realization helped him put his work into a context that made sense for him. And he had a passion for working the markets, for buying and selling, for spotting deals and

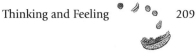

taking aggressive action. To Christopher, this was a life filled with color, emotion and fun.

Using these emotions, connecting them with his ideas, with his thoughts, Christopher established balance in his life. He established a fluid natural balance of thinking and feeling. And as he did, his life began to make sense.

How Do You Lose the Balance of Emotion and Thought?

In the previous chapters, you have seen the ways that modern life disturbs your brain's natural balance. Where the natural path of being with people is to relate in depth to a small group of people, in modern life you relate to vast numbers of people in a superficial and stimulating manner. Where the natural path to health involves vigorous exercise and daily rhythmic movement, in modern life you sit and watch as the tension builds. Where the natural path to understanding life involves creating a personal narrative to guide your behavior, in modern life you are flooded by rapid-fire stimulation that overwhelms your ability to comprehend, pulling you into a worried, contingent style of life. Where the healthy balance of appetites involves planning and delay, to find the resources to satisfy, in modern life you can consume at will and never have to plan.

This table describes these issues for you:

paths to natural balance	balance problems in modern life
close relationships with a small group of people	superficial contact with vast numbers of people
vigorous exercise and rhythmic movement	sitting still; tension rises
following a personal story based on natural skills	flooded by data and alone; pulled to the moment; alone with worry and doubt
abstinence and planning help you find resources	consume at will; no planning necessary

It is not a pretty picture. As you pursue the passion of modern life, as you take advantage of the richness and possibility of modern life, you lose balance. And it is a problem that builds on itself.

In order to live with a balance of emotion and thought, a balance of thinking and feeling, you must have close relationships with people; you must be able to move so you can process your thoughts and feelings; you must have a sense of who you are and what you are good at; and you must understand and plan for your needs.

Why? Because that is how your brain works in balance. The energy of your mind is processed and directed through your interactions with people, through movement, through your identity and your skills, and through the energy of your physical needs. The balance of emotion and thought is the result. Lacking balance in these areas means there is no way to balance emotion and thought. No way. You cannot balance emotion and thought in the abstract. You cannot balance emotion and thought alone. You cannot balance emotion and thought if you have no needs. And you cannot balance emotion and thought if you are uncertain of your story, if you are uncertain who you are.

Modern Life Separates Thinking from Feeling

As you sit in your car or on the bus, as you sit at home watching television or working at the computer, you are immobile, alone, flooded and overstimulated; emotion is inexorably separated from thought. It is just not possible to process your thoughts and your emotions when you are sitting still, by yourself, eating junk food. You can certainly think. Legions of college students studying for exams in just this way would attest to that fact. And you can certainly experience emotion, induced artificially by the wonders of the media. What you cannot do is achieve a balance of emotion and thought.

For many reasons, in Western culture, the incorrect notion that thinking is separate from feeling has taken a firm hold. The separation of mind and body, also called the pursuit of reason, has been wonderfully productive for humankind. This philosophy is responsible for the advances in technology and the improvement in the quality of life from which we all benefit.

This philosophy is powerful. It is productive. It has

become a central belief of culture in the Western world. Almost without question, we accept the notion that mind and body are separate, that emotion and intellect are different worlds of experience.

While the pursuit of reason is good for science and technology, it is not good for the pursuit of balance. This successful philosophy has interfered with the natural human path to balance, replacing it with an unnatural split between thinking and feeling.

You spend your day awash in a sea of intellectual stimulation, of facts and figures, of machines that process information at a rapid pace, of an endless succession of thoughtful analysis, of forms and procedures, of computer software, of new time-saving, thought-demanding gadgets. There is a compelling drive to be rational, logical and analytic. It is just not possible to interact with modern devices without divorcing yourself from emotion. Who among us has not experienced the helpless anger caused by a mistake we made with the VCR, or the ATM or the microwave or even trying to park our cars? Mistakes that happen because you are sad or worried, or angry or filled with love after leaving your mate. Interact with modern gadgets at your peril, if you are filled with emotion. To live today, you are forced to separate emotion from your thoughts so that you can interact with the impersonal world of technology and machines.

Bureaucracy, a type of technology that impacts us every day, is a technology where the separation of thinking and feeling has been perfected. When you become a number, a set of forms, subject to policies and procedures, you are

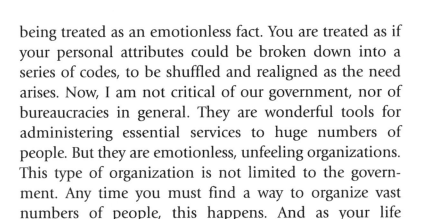

being treated as an emotionless fact. You are treated as if your personal attributes could be broken down into a series of codes, to be shuffled and realigned as the need arises. Now, I am not critical of our government, nor of bureaucracies in general. They are wonderful tools for administering essential services to huge numbers of people. But they are emotionless, unfeeling organizations. This type of organization is not limited to the government. Any time you must find a way to organize vast numbers of people, this happens. And as your life becomes involved with large bureaucratic organizations, you deal with cold facts and numbers. You lose emotion.

But we crave emotion. Feeling emotion is a basic human need. Without emotion, you wither and die. And so we have used the same wonderful technologies to produce a world of artificial emotion for our entertainment: drama, excitement, lust, tragedy, sadness, produced for us so that we can feel something. It certainly stimulates feeling deep within the lower centers of your brain. But it is feeling without meaning. It is feeling totally unconnected to whom we are; unconnected to our thoughts and values, unconnected to our skills and preferences, unconnected to people we care about. Because it lacks meaning, it is deeply unsatisfying. So we try a little harder, and our entertainments become more and more emotionally stimulating with each passing year. Clever people are working every day in the entertainment industry, to try and deliver emotion-packed entertainment because we crave it.

Here is a quote from James Gleick, in *Faster*, to illustrate the point.

We don't get scared when a commercial for Nike or Pepsi goes off on our screen like a string of firecrackers, but still, how much do we comprehend? How do we feel afterward? What will we want to do next? Reviewers talk routinely now about visual candy and visual popcorn, of the sinews of plot and character melting away in a boil of visceral gratification.

Consider that our need for emotion is so great, that it drives us to greater and greater lengths to achieve an emotional thrill, that we now routinely entertain ourselves with activities that are dangerous. We skydive, hang from kites, jump out of planes, race cars. We take dangerous drugs like cocaine and ecstasy trying to enhance emotional involvement. We go whitewater rafting, climb mountains, scuba dive in impossible places. We even bungee jump, tying a rubber band around our legs, hurtling off of bridges and cranes for the thrill of a death-defying experience. Our need for emotional experience is everywhere you look.

Consider this headline from the *Boston Globe:* "Bigger, faster [roller]-coasters tied to head injuries. Findings in new study alarming, doctors say."

And it is all out of balance. No matter how big the thrill, how nonstop the action, it is not right. It is not satisfying. It is emotion, taken out of context, artificial and devoid of meaning.

This quote from movie critic Anthony Lane in *Faster* says it all: ". . . our own ever-growing predicament: there

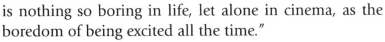

is nothing so boring in life, let alone in cinema, as the boredom of being excited all the time."

Almost everything about modern life is cerebral, engaging your thinking, your intellect in challenging and exhausting ways. At the same time, you are flooded with artificial forms of emotional excitement and stimulation. And because of the ways that modern life interferes with natural balance, thinking is separate from feeling.

What happens to you in this circumstance? What happens when you think without feeling and feel without thinking?

You lose balance. Thinking that is separated from feeling can become dull and lifeless. You lose motivation and any sense of reward for your activities. Your thoughts become lost in a stream of facts, figures, forms and analysis. Life becomes one more owner's manual to decipher, one more appliance to figure out, one more computer program to have to learn. It is deadening, exhausting and overwhelming.

Yet, to your brain it is alarming. Because your brain developed in ancient times to help we humans to survive, lower levels of your brain apply an emotional meaning to your thoughts. When you live with an endless stream of intellectual challenge, your brain interprets this as a cause for alarm. In the patterns of instinctive thought, unleashed by the separation of emotion from thought, your brain decides that there is danger in the world, and that is why your intellect is working so hard.

As you become lost in the intellectual challenges of modern life, your brain automatically starts to worry. You become stressed, anxious and easily upset by the smallest detail. Why? Because the lower centers of your brain are constantly telling you to watch out.

Even though emotionless thought can cause you to feel lifeless, apathetic and overwhelmed, at the same time, because of the instinctive reactions of your lower brain centers, you become agitated, worried and easily angered about things going wrong.

In a strange paradox of modern life, our forms of entertainment compound this situation. Exposed endlessly to artificially enhanced, thoughtless emotion, we become charged with emotional energy that has no meaning. Each time you experience the high emotional drama that is abundantly available in the entertainment world, your brain becomes even more anxious, edgy and alarmed.

It all produces the strange modern syndrome of lifeless, demoralized apathy combined with hair-trigger rage at the slightest inconvenience. You could see this at work in the story about Christopher.

Consider these facts that testify to this paradoxical syndrome:

1. The incidence of depression has been steadily rising in the past one hundred years. In cultures where it has been measured, the rates of depression increase, as Western-style technologies are adopted. Suicide among adolescents is at epidemic levels. As technology squeezes all of the emotion out of day-to-day life, we become lifeless, flattened, depressed.

2. Workplace and school violence is becoming commonplace. Just in the past couple of years alone,

there have been mass killings in Littleton, Colorado; in Wakefield, Massachusetts; in Seattle, Washington; in Miami, Florida; in Kentucky. The mentally challenging but emotionally barren settings in work and school have become a breeding ground for violence. Emotion, suppressed and ignored, eventually erupts.

3. Road rage, air rage, store rage and desk rage are now routine parts of life. In situations where we are expected to be as much a part of a human machine as possible, in airplanes, driving a car, in crowded stores, at work, emotion can break through, in outbursts of indignant rage. In fact, the *Wall Street Journal* of January 26, 2001 provides a primer on desk rage that poses this dilemma: "Warning signs. How can you tell if a colleague has reached the breaking point?"

4. Threats of violence, extreme opinions, hateful discourse are the scourge of the Internet. In this, the most abstract and mind-based of media, unregulated and uncivil bursts of emotion are routine. Using the Internet, you are alone with your thoughts, unable to naturally process emotion. People are so unmodulated, instinctive feeling pushes through.

One way to lessen the impact of this syndrome is balance, to reestablish a healthy and harmonious balance between thought and emotion, to live in a fluid rhythm where feeling is connected with thinking. You can. We humans were able to do so for millions of years. The science proves it; the balance of thinking and feeling is the natural way that your brain operates. By following some rules of balance, you can discover your own unique balance of emotion and thought. Here is a story to illustrate the way that this is done.

Fighting Suicidal Thoughts

When we first began to work together, suicide was never far from Martha's thoughts. Criticized by her family for her temper and her negativity, angered over her husband's thoughtlessness and by the way that he did not listen to her, hopeless about her daughter's alcohol problem, bored by repetitive detail and flooded by paperwork, her job a mind-numbing nightmare researching tedious details and writing research studies for her company, Martha could not see any other way out. Suicide. In Martha's mind, it meant release. In her mind, it was the only solution for her countless problems.

Thankfully, being a religious person, Martha never accepted suicide as something she could do. Yet the feeling remained, and the idea of suicide became an unwanted focus, another burden in her life.

"I like my work," she said. "There is just too much of it. And I'm slow. I chase every detail because they are all so interesting to me. But I don't finish on time, and I get overwhelmed. Then I just want to give up."

Devoted to her children, a talented researcher, Martha had been able to create a job that allowed her to work while the kids were at school. She was senior researcher for a small biotechnology company. She was responsible for writing research protocols.

"My boss is always on me to produce more," she explained.

"The pressure really gets to me. I would go faster if I could, but I can't. He's frustrated, I'm frustrated. The lab is very tense. Sometimes I even blow my stack at him. He seems to accept it as part of who I am. I can't believe that I still have the job."

Blessed with a quick, analytic mind, Martha was a good scientist, who could develop brilliant research designs to benefit her company. But she was slow and independent-minded. She pursued each scientific issue until she had covered every angle, until she had researched every question.

"It's not sensible," she said. "Some of the scientific questions are trivial, but I just can't let go."

With her strong emotions and quick temper, traits she had struggled with since childhood, she had become very hard on herself, constantly angry with herself for what she perceived as her own failings.

This carried over to her home life. Much to her own regret, Martha yelled constantly at her husband and at her kids. Martha could not overlook any of the small details, from the crumbs that her kids left on the kitchen counter to the work messages for her husband on their home answering machine— it all bothered her.

She certainly could not overlook her daughter's trouble with alcohol. Nikki had fallen in with a bad crowd. She drank too much. When emotions were too intense at home, when Martha was angrily critical towards her, Nikki went out with her friends and drank. Her grades were poor. She was in debt. She had already lost her license. Nikki was in serious trouble. So Martha spent countless hours researching treatment programs, therapists and schools for Nikki. And it did not help. Nikki resisted and went her own way.

And then there was politics. Her husband, a civic-minded man, had been elected to the school committee. Edward insisted that Martha come with him to community fundraisers, to political dinners and to meetings of the state Republican party. It was stimulating, but it was too much.

Confronted daily by one challenging situation after another, Martha found herself angry and frustrated. Brimming with the emotional intensity that she had always felt, Martha lashed out at everyone. It only made her feel worse.

Martha's life was out of balance.

Given the strength of her emotions and her spirited personality, it made sense to us to begin a program of balance by finding ways to manage her emotions.

"If I could just find a way to be less sensitive, that would be half the battle," Martha admitted.

Raised by the seashore, when Martha worked with me to pick her tools, she found that activities related to water came naturally to her. Swimming, boating, spending a hot summer's day lying on a float in her pool, these activities made sense to her. We turned her preferences into some rules, to help her to quiet her emotions.

Martha's Rules for Managing Emotions

1. Take a hot bath in the evening to dissolve the tension of the day.
2. Use swimming as a form of rhythmic movement to help with emotional processing.

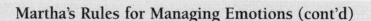

Martha's Rules for Managing Emotions (cont'd)

Another one of Martha's tools was that she liked to talk things through with people. In her present non-stop life, she had fallen out of the habit of talking things through. Instead she would just react. This led to a third rule for managing emotion, one that helped her by providing a structure, a time and a place for dealing with emotion.

3. *Instead of reacting, agree to meet for a few minutes to talk matters over. With her husband, this rule turned into a regular weekly meeting. At work, it evolved into a daily fifteen-minute meeting with her boss. And with Nikki, Martha replaced frantic phone calls, demands and arguments with regular talks at a local coffee shop, a place loved by both Martha and Nikki.*

Once Martha gained some confidence in managing her emotions, the next step was to help Martha make some decisions. Drawn in many directions at once, her life was filled with a never-ending succession of important matters. No matter where she was or who she was with, there were challenges and demands for her to address.

"This is all my doing," she said. "If I wasn't so ambitious, maybe I would have just stayed home with the kids and been all right." But Martha was wrong. The problem was not that she was ambitious; the problem

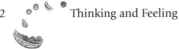

was that she was out of balance. She was lost in a world of intellectual challenge, with nothing to guide her and no way of knowing where and why to focus her energy.

To help her to figure this out, I asked Martha to complete a chart of her life.

To complete the chart, Martha reviewed key years in her life, recalling an event that she felt was important at the time. Then Martha described the emotion and rated the strength of the emotion on this scale: just a little, somewhat strongly, very strongly, powerfully, with great intensity.

Martha's life chart

Age	Life Event	Main Emotion	Intensity of Emotion
6	learning to swim	pride	somewhat strongly
13	award for biology paper	creative joy	powerfully
18	first boyfriend	love and sexual excitement	with great intensity
25	marriage	joy, love, caring	with great intensity
27	purchased first home	protective feelings, pride, joy of ownership	powerfully
28	Nikki born	joy, love, caring	with great intensity
34	finished Ph.D.	pride, accomplishment	very strongly
35	first research job	accomplishment, feeling like a contributor	somewhat strongly
40	Mom's death	grief, protective feelings	with great intensity

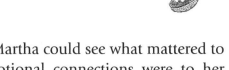

From her life chart, Martha could see what mattered to her. Her strongest emotional connections were to her family, her home and to creativity. Work and being active seemed to matter, but less so.

"I never really thought about what mattered to me," Martha said. "I can see why this is important." From this exercise, we were able to list what mattered to Martha.

What mattered to Martha:

- taking care of her family
- having a loving relationship
- creative use of her mind

These were the paths of balance for Martha. When engaged in these activities, she felt in tune with her emotions, in a harmonious balance of thought and feeling.

"I can see the problem," she told me sadly, "I don't spend enough time doing what matters to me. I spend most of my time reacting, or doing things that matter more to other people."

That led to the next step, the next rule of balance. Martha needed to find a way to become involved with things that mattered. As we talked, it became clear that her relationship with Nikki was important and also neglected. Martha had spent so much time doing and reacting that the relationship had languished and soured. She decided to spend her energy on improving the relationship with Nikki. Martha planned a week-long trip, just for the two of them, to go shopping in New York. On the trip they talked; they aired their feelings; they made plans to do things differently. With the tools for managing her emotions in place, Martha was able to work with Nikki, to soothe her, to come to a new understanding.

Next, she decided that her relationship with her husband needed to be addressed. Knowing how much he loved to sail, she proposed that they buy a small sailboat. She knew just the one, had researched it thoroughly; it was in a neighbor's yard and could be had for little expense. Understanding that activities with water were calming to her, Martha's plan was to spend time sailing with Edward, alone, with time to talk.

The last problem to solve was work. Martha now realized that being a successful research scientist was not that important. What mattered to her was to provide for her family, hopefully in a way that allowed her to think creatively. Martha worked out a plan where she could be paid as a consultant and, in that way, be better able to control her hours. Next, she developed a working relationship with a research assistant, who was delighted to have the work of writing research studies. Martha focused her efforts on creating new projects that helped her company, leaving the task of the time-consuming research to her associate. Martha ended up making a little less money, but the work became much, much more satisfying to her.

So Martha found balance by following her own rules. Martha found a way to manage her emotions. She found out what mattered, and she used these tools to help her solve some problems. That is how she found her balance.

Finding the Balance of Thinking and Feeling

To find a natural balance of emotion and thought, it is helpful to recall just what emotion was meant to do for us. In the wiring of your brain, emotion is energy that powers meaning and that powers memory. You remember important people and events because of the emotional energy generated by the encounter. And it is the energy that drives reasoning, planning and problem solving. When powered by emotion, your brain naturally searches for a reason why; your brain hungers for an explanation; your brain becomes driven to look for a solution to whatever it is that is causing you to have such strong feelings.

That is why so much of modern life is so addictive. The images, the intensity, the manufactured emotion of modern life produces strong feelings, artificially, and your poor ancient brain is compelled to remember and to make sense of it.

So far, we have talked about what we do and how we do it. Now, with the subject of mental energy, from emotion, and to a lesser extent from appetite, we talk about why. *Why?* The answer is the meaning and importance of our actions. Ultimately that is the balance of emotion and thought. To provide meaning and purpose to life. And it is through the activities that are meaningful that emotion comes to life. Activities powered by emotion become the expression of that emotion.

What does this mean? For Martha it meant that contract work, which was not meaningful, was lifeless and dull. It meant that time spent with her daughter was deeply satisfying. It meant that the simple exercise of sailing with her husband was a powerfully felt expression of her love. When emotion is linked with thought, the activities that result are comforting, satisfying and rewarding. For Christopher it meant that working and making money was methodical and deadening to his soul until he learned to link his work to activities that meant something to him. When he understood that the money he made at work could help him build a relationship with his daughter, work became more meaningful. When he could see how to take his money and use it to create a hobby business that was a source of reward and pleasure for him, then work was infused with energy, with meaning, with emotion.

Since modern life has effectively unlinked thinking and feeling, since we have become driven by information separate from emotion, this natural process of balance has been interrupted. Feeling, detached from thought and from purposeful activity, becomes an unregulated visceral function, much like an appetite. As is true for the balance problems we have seen with appetite, the excitement, the abundance, the richness of modern life leads to emotional stimulation, to unregulated emotionality, to peaks and valleys of emotions that are not soothed and processed by actions that make sense. When you unlink feeling from thought, as modern life does, then there is nothing to naturally regulate, structure, time or *conduct* the flow of your emotions. That becomes the focus of some natural rules for balancing feeling and thinking.

Like appetite, emotion is an energy source for your mind. Like appetite, the first rules of balance have to do with managing your emotion. By this I mean learning ways to time, structure, regulate and soothe your emotional energy in much the same way that this would happen naturally, in the past. By managing your emotions, I mean learning to create conditions that mimic the flow of emotion that would occur if your emotions were fluidly linked to thinking and action; to people in your life; to movement; to problem solving and planning; to the memory of important events. Emotion and thought in balance.

When thinking and feeling work in balance, your emotion is discharged smoothly as you act and think. In modern life, this link is broken, so your day is spent thinking and reacting, or your emotions are powerfully discharged through the drama of the entertainment world. This can leave you tense, over stimulated and ready to explode over the smallest matter. This leads to some natural rules for balancing thinking and feeling.

Rule #1: Learn to Soothe Yourself and to Reduce Built-Up Tension

How can you do this? There are as many ways as there are people. What works is any activity that is relaxing, soothing and calming. Almost everyone knows a way to do this for themselves, the real trick is taking the time to do it. Here are some common ways that people soothe and calm themselves:

- exercise
- hot baths

- listening to quiet music
- playing an instrument
- talking with a supportive person
- meditation
- yoga
- reading

Almost any quiet, rhythmic and peaceful activity will do. I like to reduce my tension through swimming, gardening and reading. A woman I know relaxes by cleaning the house. Christopher painted landscapes to calm himself.

It could be anything. You will need about fifteen to thirty minutes to calm yourself effectively. Then you will be ready to go at it again.

Rule #2: Pay Attention to the Structure of Your Emotions: The Timing and Rhythm

Try not to solve the unsolvable. By flooding you with nonstop intellectual challenge, modern life can cause you to try and solve problems that are unsolvable. If everything is urgent and immediate, you can be drawn into a driven, compulsive search for answers—even when there are none to be had. You see, the nonstop pace of modern life captivates our simple-minded ancient brains. Your brain reacts as if a herd of elephants were charging your village all of the time!

But emotions do not work that way. There is a flow to the balance of emotion and thought, with peaks and valleys

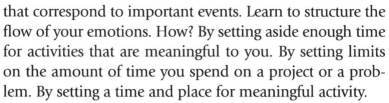

that correspond to important events. Learn to structure the flow of your emotions. How? By setting aside enough time for activities that are meaningful to you. By setting limits on the amount of time you spend on a project or a problem. By setting a time and place for meaningful activity.

A good general rule to follow is the ninety-minute rule. The rhythm of your brain is such that you can only be effectively involved with a meaningful activity for about ninety minutes at a time. Then you need a break. Longer than ninety minutes and the tension starts to build.

Another good rule to follow is the "can I think about it" rule. Since much of the time you are immobile and pre-occupied with thought, you are not really in a mode that is conducive to processing emotion and thought. If you are presented with a situation that has an emotional impact, give yourself time and the proper tools to think about it. It is just not physically possible to process thought and emotion quickly while you are sitting still. Your brain needs time and movement to think.

And the energy to link thinking and feeling is not always available on demand, as much as we would like it to be. Emotional energy, like the energy of your appetites, waxes and wanes depending on your circumstance. If you are not receptive, then it just won't work. Find out what your rhythms are and live within them. Is your emotional energy higher in the morning? Or at night? At the beginning of the week, or at the end? Is your emotional energy higher when you are with a group of people, or one-on-one?

Rule #3: Move Rhythmically

As you saw in the chapter on movement, rhythmic movement helps your brain to process thinking and feeling. Be sure that there is enough rhythmic movement in your life and you will find it easier to balance emotion and thought.

Rule #4: Connect Thinking and Feeling by Using Your Tools

Your tools are those activities that are naturally suited to who you are. Refer back to the chapter on the balance of past and present to better understand how you pick your tools.

When you use your tools, there will be a natural rhythm and flow linking your thoughts and your feelings. Your behavioral tools are the pathway that your brain uses to tie emotion and thought together. In the workings of your mind, emotion and thought will tell you *why* you are using your tools. Emotion and thought link up by providing a reason for your actions, the energy to use your tools. When emotion and thought are in balance, you have energy, motivation and a reason to act. Then your behavioral tools tell you *what to* do and *how to* do it. Your unique set of behavior tools become the living and breathing expression of the meaning provided by emotion and thought. When you are using your unique set of behavioral tools, you are letting your mind and brain work in the way that it was created, with a natural and fluid linkage between thought, feeling and action.

Since your nervous system is a two-way street, as you use your tools, you sense this (actually your right brain senses this) and it feels right. As you link emotion, feeling and action together, in a way that makes sense, your mind takes notice; performing an emotionally meaningful activity, using your natural skills, just feels good. It is a boost to your confidence to be true to yourself in a way that has meaning.

No matter how your life is put together, make sure that you spend time using your repertoire of behavioral tools. When you do so, you will have a natural path toward feeling confident satisfaction in your day.

Once you have confidence in your ability to manage the emotional overflow from everyday life, then it is time to consider what really matters to you. One way of understanding the balance of emotion and thought is that it provides the *why*, for what you do. The directed energy that you will feel when emotion and thought are in balance can be used by you as a source of motivation, enthusiasm and meaning for your life. When you have a balance of thinking and feeling, you will be better able to prioritize, to make decisions, to take action and solve problems. You will be confident that you understand *why*. The *why* of things leads us to the next natural rule for balancing thinking and feeling.

Rule #5: Find Out What Really Matters to You

You can discover what matters to you by looking into your own history to track important events—times when you had strong feelings, situations that felt powerful. The secret here is that you will remember the events that matter because of the emotion you felt. Remember, emotional energy powers memory. Powerful or significant events are vivid in your mind because they were emotionally important and because these events represented the manner in which emotion and thought interact for you.

There is a secret to this exercise. There are key times in life when emotional learning crystalizes. Because of the way the brain develops, there are phases in life when emotion and thought come together, forming patterns of understanding that you will use for the rest of your life. In part because of the influence of your upbringing, in part because of the circumstances of your life, in part because of the emotional wiring that you inherited, when you pass through these important phases, your mind and brain create an understanding of life that blends emotion and thought into one. These key, developmental phases are summarized on following page.

Review your life, especially during these key times. Try to recall important events and the feeling associated with these events. Understand how you felt as part of the experience. Ask yourself, "How did I feel during those times?" "What turned me on?" "Was I sad, satisfied, proud or excited?" "Was I feeling accomplished, rewarded or gratified?" Take a hard look at who you were with, at what you were doing, at the flow of your day-to-day life. That will tell you how thinking and feeling are blended

Key Times in Life

Age	What You Learn
4 to 6	How to get along with others
11 to 13	Living with your unique attributes; living with demands from others
17 to 20	Becoming an individual, separate from but in tune with other people
20 to 30	How to establish a place in the world for you and your family. Being a parent
40 to 50	Understanding the natural limits of life. Being alone in the world as your elders pass on
55 to 65	How to help others grow and prosper
65 to 80	Coming to terms with the nature of your life. Wisdom. The importance of continuity

for you. That will tell you what really matters. Here are some ideas for prompting your memory:

- Look at old photographs and videos.
- Talk with older members of your family to get their view of you at these times.
- Talk with a therapist. (This collecting of memories is a key component of most therapies.)

- Take a trip to the places you lived during these times.
- Take out your souvenirs and momentos; look at them and remember.

As you review your history, you will get a sense of what mattered to you. When you are done, keep a record of the people and activities that mattered paired with a record of how you felt.

Then, when you are done, make a life chart, like the one that Martha made, as a record of what really matters to you. Simply having the knowledge of what matters to you is a powerful tool of balance. When you know how thinking and feeling come together for you in action, it will provide guidance for your life; it will provide confidence that you are doing the right thing.

Putting Your Emotional Energy to Work

The grand plan, the great scheme, what mattered most for millions of years was survival. The wonderful mechanisms of your mind were created to be certain that you survived. The linkage of emotion, thought and action is the natural pathway for this to happen. Our ancestors took action, and remembered what worked because of how they felt: the warmth and sensual pleasures of family life, the pride and satisfaction of a successful hunt, the pleasure and security of helping other members of the village. In each circumstance, emotion and thought came together into actions that sustained life. Each day was filled with actions that solved the central problem of how to survive another day.

Today, of course, that is not true. For most of us, survival is not at issue. We are well-fed, well-cared for, abundantly entertained. Our ancient brains no longer have to use the energy of emotion and thought to allow us to survive. Today, emotion is something you feel at the movies or on a roller-coaster. Thought and intellectual demand is what floods us each and every day.

To find balance, you must reunite thinking, feeling and action. As was true for our ancestors, you will feel best when you are doing what matters most, when you have an emotional and intellectual investment. How can you do this? By using your heart and your mind to handle a challenge in life that really matters. As if it were necessary to survive. Link up your thinking and your feeling with a plan of action that matters to you. That is the last step on the path to balance for emotions and thought. The last rule is:

Rule #6: Make a Plan to Take Action

Focus on the areas that matter, the parts of life that have an emotional impact on you. Look to your life chart. You'll see. Is it making money? Is it raising a family? Is it being the best at something? Is it the act of creating? Is it forming relationships? Take what matters to you and create a plan to make it better. Not just to survive, but to flourish. Use your heart and your mind to find the energy, the motivation, the *reward* in life. That is the essence of this step.

Martha solved the problem of how to be a better parent to her daughter because caring for her family, being a good mom, really mattered to her. She solved the problem of how to make work more rewarding by finding a way to be creative. Being creative with her mind really mattered.

Christopher found a way to enjoy life more by understanding the pleasure and pride that making money brought to him. It really mattered to him that he made a lot of money because of the way he could use that money to bring enjoyment to him and his daughter.

Here are some ideas that you can use to reunite thinking and feeling to help you to take action on what really matters to you.

- **Catch yourself doing things right:** When you are working on what matters, take time to notice what went well, what pleased you and what you feel good about. The natural inclination is to be self-critical and then that is what you recall. But if instead you consciously compliment yourself as you are working on what matters, then you will recall a good feeling when you remember what you did.

- **Savor the emotional rewards:** After you have done a task, take some time to reflect on the positive emotion that you felt. Instead of focusing on the next thing to be done, savor the warmth of love you felt with your children; savor the pride of accomplishment when you completed a project; savor excitement and fun of playing tennis with your best friend. Taking action on what matters to you will generate these positive emotions. Savor them, remember them, use the positive energy they provide.

- **Keep reminders of what matters:** Pictures, videos, cards and keepsakes are powerful tools to prompt your memory to recall positive emotions. Be sure to keep reminders of the times when you felt a flowing rhythm of emotion and thought, when you were doing what mattered. Then, when you are feeling stressed, tense or blue, take out your pictures, watch your videos, look at your cards and souvenirs. They will evoke the memories of the positive flow of emotion and action that you cherish.

- **Tell stories:** There is no better way to help yourself take action on what really matters, to reinforce the power of your emotions, to balance thinking and feeling, than by telling stories. This uniquely human activity engages your brain, your mind and your heart. Tell stories to your children, to your mate, to your friends and colleagues. It will lighten your heart. It will energize you to keep going. It will help you be sure of your plan, be more confident of your actions. It will help you recapture the deep satisfaction that comes when you combine thinking, feeling and action.

The Balance of Thinking and Feeling

There is a flowing energy to life that comes from emotion. Tap into this energy. Use it for motivation, for pleasure and for a confident sense of what to do. Understand what matters to you; focus your actions in a way that makes sense for who you are. Link your feelings and your thoughts into fluid and purposeful action. Our brains were created to work that way.

Thinking and Feeling Self-Test

Take this test to see if you are out of balance. If you answered yes to two or more questions, then you may have a problems with the balance of past and present. To improve your balance, to incorporate the rules in this chapter as well as the tips to follow.

1. Do the circumstances of your life often cause you to feel demoralized, apathetic or lifeless?　　　　　　　　　　　　　　yes　　　no
2. Do you find yourself feeling tense, angry or impatient over insignificant details like waiting in line?　　　　　　　　　　yes　　　no
3. Do you find yourself drawn to activities that provide high levels of excitement or emotional stimulation?　　　　　　　yes　　　no
4. Do you often find yourself confused about the purpose and meaning of your life?　yes　　　no

Score _____

Tips to Balance Thinking and Feeling

Here is a list of tips to help put your natural rules to work for you.

Try incorporating some of these tips each week of your balance program. When you do, you will be on the way to creating a meaningful balance of thinking and feeling in your life.

1. Stretch your muscles. At the end of a long day, try stretching to relieve the emotional tension that has built up in your body throughout the day. All of the nonstop intellectual demand of today's information age can leave you tense and overstimulated. Stretching is a natural antidote for this problem. Stretching is simple, easy and effective at reducing nervous tension. Pair stretching with rhythmic breathing and you have a powerful stress reduction tool. All for free!

2. Try fidgeting. Whenever you must complete a task that is intellectually challenging and emotionally unrewarding—tasks like doing your taxes or paying bills, or writing a résumé, or filling out insurance paperwork, or watching political debates on TV—try fidgeting. You could doodle or play with paper clips. You could play with one of those ingenious desk-top toys whose purpose is simply to give you an outlet for your nervous energy. When you fidget, you are using your hands to provide an outlet for the nervous stimulation that results from an intellectually demanding, but emotionally unrewarding activity. Fidgeting can release tension and by doing so, it can help you to focus on your task.

3. Make a habit of saying "Can I think about it?" Our ancient brains need time to balance thinking and feeling. Reacting on the spot, while satisfying, can lead you to decisions that make you unhappy. Take

time to think. Move about, relax. Let the natural processes of your brain work to link thinking and feeling. Once you understand the emotional and intellectual dimensions of a particular circumstance, then make your decision.

4. Use sleep to connect thinking and feeling. Troubled by an unsolvable problem? Can't make up your mind? Not sure what to do? Try sleeping on it. What seems confusing and unsolvable at 2 A.M., can magically be clear and direct after a refreshing night's sleep. As you sleep, your mind is working to link thinking and feeling. As you sleep, your brain makes connections—memories, patterns of thought, emotional and creative insights. Your brain does this by actually linking different parts of your brain together in patterns of nerve cell excitation. Relax your thoughts and go to sleep. Let your brain do its job of linking thinking and feeling through the healing processes of sleep.

5. Use the chart on page 233 as a guide to reviewing your life. Try to recall important events, and the feeling associated with these events. Understand how you felt as part of the experience. Ask yourself, "How did I feel during those times?" "What turned me on?" "Was I sad, satisfied, proud or excited?" "Was I feeling accomplished, rewarded or gratified?" Take a hard look at who you were with; at what you were doing; at the flow of your day-to-day life. Your review will tell you how thinking and feeling are blended for you into life events that really matter.

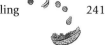

6. Make a plan that uses your skills; do what works for you. Once you have a clear sense of what has worked for you in the past—what activities, interests or relationships filled you with passion and purpose—make a plan to put these skills to work. For example, if music gets you going, then use it to solve a problem. Take your child to a concert and while you are there, talk a little bit about their homework problems. Do you love to cook? Then broaden your social life by inviting friends over for dinner. Are you a people person? Then help yourself to deal with all of the time in the car by getting a cell phone and making calls to friends and family while you sit in traffic. Are you good at handling money and numbers? Then plan to go back to school for a business degree, once your children are older.

7. Hang your awards, certificates, diplomas and photographs of celebrations on the wall. Even if you never finished school you more than likely have special belongings that serve the purpose of diplomas. These momentos are concrete symbols of what went right for you. They help you to remember those times when you were filled with passion and purpose, when your thinking and feeling flowed in a natural balance. These special possessions include photos, awards, plaques, small figures, religious symbols, things that you have made and many other items that carry this special meaning for you.

   Find them and hang them on the wall. And as

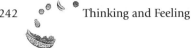

you look at these special belongings take pride in your accomplishment. Renew your sense of what matters and what works for you.

8. Remember your role models. Talk to them if you can. Role models are key figures who have a deep influence on who you are. Parents, teachers, coaches, clergymen, or prominent public people like politicians can all serve as role models. As you pattern yourself after a role model, your brain naturally connects thinking and feeling into purposeful activity. When you follow the example of your role model, your right brain blends an understanding of their skills with an emotional connection. The result is a skill set for you that produces a confident sense of who you are and what to do.

   Remember your role models. If you can, talk with them, watch them in action, renew the memories of their influence on you.

9. Use the tips about movement from chapter 4. All of the tips about movement can work to help you to calm, soothe and quiet the nervous tension that builds up every day. Use them to calm your nerves. When you do, you will be better able to create a natural balance of thinking and feeling.

10. Keep track of your feelings. What turned you on? What made you sad? What bored you to tears? Who do you like? Who helps you to feel confident? All day long your brain and your heart react with feeling. Learn to keep track of these feelings and to the thoughts, actions and people

associated with them. This will help you to link thinking and feeling so that you develop a better sense of what matters to you. Over time you will see patterns in your behavior, patterns in your reactions. You can use this understanding to fill your day-to-day life with passion and purpose.

There are many ways to do this. No one method is the "right" method. Some people remember words and conversations. Some remember images. Some keep a list. Some rely on feedback from others. Try different approaches until you find the right one for you.

READER/CUSTOMER CARE SURVEY

BB1

We care about your opinions. Please take a moment to fill out this Reader Survey card and mail it back to us.
As a special **"thank you"** we'll send you exciting news about interesting books and a valuable **Gift Certificate.**

Please PRINT using ALL CAPS

First Name		MI.	Last Name

Address

City		ST	Zip

Phone # (| | |) | | | | — | | | | |

Email

(1) Gender:
___ Female   ___ Male

(2) Age:
___ 12 or under   ___ 40-59
___ 13-19   ___ 60+
___ 20-39

(3) Marital Status
___ Married
___ Single
___ Divorced/Widowed

(4) Did you receive this book as a gift?
___ Yes   ___ No

(5) How many Health Communications books have you bought or read?
___ 1   ___ 2-4   ___ 5+

(6) How did you find out about this book?
Please fill in ONE.
1) ___ Recommendation
2) ___ Store Display
3) ___ Bestseller List
4) ___ Online
5) ___ Advertisement
6) ___ Catalog/Mailing
7) ___ Interview/Review (TV, Radio, Print)

(7) Where do you usually buy books?
Please fill in your top TWO choices.
1) ___ Bookstore
2) ___ Religious Bookstore
3) ___ Online
4) ___ Book Club/Mail Order
5) ___ Price Club (Costco, Sam's Club, etc.)
6) ___ Retail Store (Target, Wal-mart, etc.)

(9) What subjects do you enjoy reading about most? Rank only *FIVE.* Use 1 for your favorite, 2 for second favorite, etc.

	1	2	3	4	5
1) Parenting/Family	○	○	○	○	○
2) Relationships	○	○	○	○	○
3) Recovery/Addictions	○	○	○	○	○
4) Health/Nutrition	○	○	○	○	○
5) Christianity	○	○	○	○	○
6) Spirituality/Inspiration	○	○	○	○	○
7) Business Self-Help	○	○	○	○	○
8) Teen Issues	○	○	○	○	○
9) Sports	○	○	○	○	○

(14) What attracts you most to a book?
(Please rank 1-4 in order of preference.)

	1	2	3	4
1) Title	○	○	○	○
2) Cover Design	○	○	○	○
3) Author	○	○	○	○
4) Content	○	○	○	○

TAPE IN MIDDLE; DO NOT STAPLE

BUSINESS REPLY MAIL

FIRST-CLASS MAIL PERMIT NO 45 DEERFIELD BEACH, FL

POSTAGE WILL BE PAID BY ADDRESSEE

HEALTH COMMUNICATIONS, INC.
3201 SW 15TH STREET
DEERFIELD BEACH FL 33442-9875

FOLD HERE

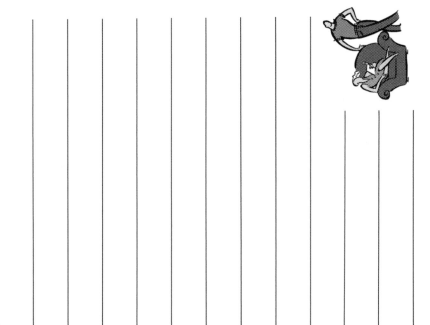

Comments:

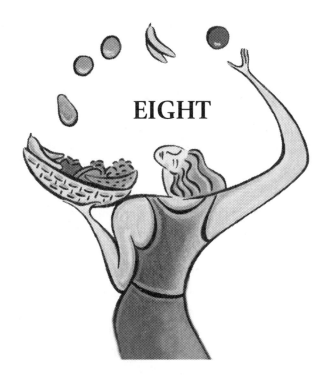

EIGHT

System 6:
Sleep and Wakefulness

Of all the practices known to be associated with
good health, sleep is the most fundamental.

J. Allan Hobson, *The Chemistry of Conscious States*

How Much Should You Sleep?

What is the right amount of sleep for you? Do you get enough healthy sleep? Do you sleep too much? These are not simple questions, as I will explain. But these are the central questions for sleep balance. Sleeping the right amount, for the needs of your body and your brain, is a natural rule of balance. Notice that I referred to sleeping the *right* amount. It is not simply a matter of getting enough sleep. Your natural rules for sleep balance are really all about getting the right amount of sleep for your particular body and brain, for your personal needs.

Consider that a single night of sleep deprivation causes you to lose 30 to 40 percent of your mental efficiency. A second night of sleep deprivation and you lose 60 to 70 percent of your mental efficiency. After only six nights of insufficient sleep, your body begins to show signs of distress. Six nights of inadequate sleep, and your thyroid is suppressed, the stress hormone, cortisol increases, and you begin to show early signs of diabetes.

We are a sleep-deprived nation. The National Commission of Sleep Disorders Research estimated that twelve years ago, in 1988, the cost of accidents related to sleepiness was over $43 billion. Circadian Information Inc., a consulting firm in Cambridge, Massachusetts, estimates that 23 million people work nights or evenings.

Sleepiness while driving is a cause of over 100,000 auto accidents per year, which result in over 1,500 deaths as reported in the *Journal of the American Medical Association*.

There is a simple biologic fact that bedevils we modern

humans. For every person, there is an amount of sleep that is right. Not too much sleep. Not too little sleep. As much as we would like to believe that sleep is something we can control—sleeping when there is time, staying up when there is something to do—this is just not the case. To live in balance you must *sleep the right amount.*

What is the right amount of sleep? It is different for each person. The amount of sleep that you need is unique for you, just as your height, your coloring and your body type is unique to you. The average sleep length for a healthy adult is between seven to eight hours per night (7.5 hours per night to be exact). Most people need around this amount of sleep. This is an average figure, and, as is true for all averages, there is also a huge variation from person to person. Some people are short sleepers, feeling energetic and alert after only three or four hours of sleep. Others are long sleepers, who don't feel alert and energized unless sleeping ten to twelve hours per night.

If you are a short sleeper, you cannot turn yourself into a long sleeper. If you are a long sleeper, you will not be able to turn yourself into a short sleeper. Sleeping the right amount—the length of sleep that is required by the physical characteristics of your brain, your body and your mind—is the first step on the path to balance. If you do not get the right amount of sleep, then you will lose your sleep balance. Then, in all likelihood, you will feel tired all of the time. What sleep you do get will be unsettled and inefficient. You may wind up in a downward spiral of dysfunction. You will not be able to live a balanced life.

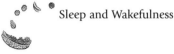

To find out if you are sleeping the right amount, answer the following questions.

1. Do you still feel tired when you get up from sleep?	yes	no
2. Do you sleep late whenever you can?	yes	no
3. Do you feel excessively sleepy during the day?	yes	no
4. Do you function better during the day if you take a nap?	yes	no
5. If you do nap, do you still feel tired after you nap?	yes	no
6. Do you have trouble staying awake during the day?	yes	no
7. Do you lie in bed awake, unable to fall asleep, causing you to oversleep in the morning?	yes	no
8. Do you sleep more than ten hours per day and still feel tired?	yes	no

If you answered yes to four or more of these questions, then you may not be sleeping for the *right* amount of time. You will have noticed that I always refer to sleeping the right amount of time. That is because your sleep can be out of balance because you are undersleeping or because you are oversleeping. Here is a description of each problem.

Undersleeping

In everyday language, this condition is commonly described as being sleep-deprived, and it is a condition familiar to all of us. If you are undersleeping you will feel tired all of the time; you will be prone to falling asleep during the day, while driving, studying or performing any routine activity; you will have more trouble concentrating and more trouble with your memory; you may notice mood changes, possibly feeling depressed and cranky. If you have been undersleeping for a long time, your health can begin to deteriorate; you may develop high blood pressure; you may catch colds, the flu and pneumonia more easily. In extreme form, undersleeping may cause you to become psychotic.

Oversleeping

This condition is less familiar to most people. The idea that oversleeping can cause problems is counterintuitive. But it can. If you are oversleeping, your sleep cycle becomes irregular and unbalanced. That is what causes the problems: Your sleep cycle becomes out of synch with the natural rhythm of night and day. If you are oversleeping you will tend to feel tired all of the time, but unlike the problems with undersleeping, you will not be prone to falling asleep during routine activities. You will have trouble falling asleep at night, and trouble getting out of bed in the morning; you may end up sleeping late into the day. Your sleep will not seem restful. You may tend to feel depressed and worried; it may be hard for you to get your mind off of your troubles. You will have trouble getting motivated; you may feel overwhelmed when you think about what you have to do. When you are awake, you may feel restless, bored and dissatisfied with your life. You will have a tendency to put on weight; you may feel that exercise is impossible and so you become physically out of shape.

You can effectively solve the riddle of how much sleep you need, and begin to structure your sleep into a healthy balance by using a simple sleep chart. People often find that the act of keeping a chart of sleep activity begins to set a healthy sleep process in motion.

Draw a sleep chart on a blank piece of paper, so that it looks like the sleep chart on page 247.

For each hour of the day put in a W, if you are awake, and an S if you are asleep.

Then on the second line marked "state" put in the code for your energy state. If you are sleeping put in an R for restful sleep or a P for poor or restless sleep. For times that you are awake, code an H for a rested or high-energy state, when you are feeling well. Code a T, for a low-energy, tired state. Then connect all of the W's, all of the S's, all of the H's and all of the T's

After you keep this chart for a week you will have a picture of when you sleep, when you are awake and how you feel during those times. Here is an example of the way that a sleep chart would look for me in a typical week. For our purposes, each day starts with the sunset of the previous day. For example, our chart for Sunday begins with sunset (7:00 P.M.) on Saturday.

Sleep Chart

	7 pm	8 pm	9 pm	10 pm	11 pm	12 pm	1 am	2 am	3 am	4 am	5 am	6 am	7 am	8 am	9 am	10 am	11 am	12 am	1 pm	2 pm	3 pm	4 pm	5 pm	6 pm

Sunday

state

Monday

state

Tuesday

state

Wednesday

state

Thursday

state

Friday

state

Saturday

state

Paul's Sleep Chart

	7 pm	8 pm	9 pm	10 pm	11 pm	12 pm	1 am	2 am	3 am	4 am	5 am	6 am	7 am	8 am	9 am	10 am	11 am	12 am	1 pm	2 pm	3 pm	4 pm	5 pm	6 pm
Sunday	w	w	w	s	s	s	s	s	s	s	s	w	w	w	w	w	w	w	w	w	w	w	w	w
state	h	t	t	r	r	r	r	r	r	r	p	h	h	h	h	h	h	h	h	h	h	h	t	t
Monday	w	w	w	w	s	s	s	s	s	s	s	w	w	w	w	w	w	w	w	w	w	w	w	h
state	t	t	t	t	r	r	r	r	r	r	p	h	h	h	h	h	h	h	h	h	h	h	h	h
Tuesday	w	w	w	s	s	s	s	s	s	s	s	w	w	w	w	w	w	w	w	w	w	w	w	w
state	t	t	t	r	r	r	r	r	r	r	p	h	h	h	h	h	h	h	h	h	h	t	t	t
Wednesday	w	w	w	w	s	s	s	s	s	s	s	w	w	w	w	w	w	w	w	w	w	w	w	w
state	h	h	t	t	r	r	r	r	r	r	p	h	h	h	h	h	h	h	h	h	h	t	t	t
Thursday	w	w	w	w	w	s	s	s	s	s	s	w	w	w	w	w	w	w	w	w	w	w	w	w
state	t	t	t	t	t	r	r	r	r	r	t	h	h	h	h	h	h	h	h	h	t	t	t	h
Friday	w	w	w	w	w	w	s	s	s	s	s	w	w	w	w	w	w	w	w	w	w	w	w	w
state	t	t	t	t	t	t	r	r	r	r	h	h	h	h	h	h	h	h	h	t	t	t	t	t
Saturday	w	w	w	w	s	s	s	s	s	s	s	s	s	s	w	w	w	w	w	w	w	w	w	w
state	t	t	t	t	r	r	r	r	t	t	t	r	p	p	t	h	h	h	t	t	t	t	t	t

From the picture provided by my sleep chart, you can see that I do best when I sleep between seven to eight hours per day. When I sleep less than this, I begin to be more tired in the afternoon and evening. You can also see that I tend to sleep less during the week when I am working, and that this fact begins to unbalance my natural sleep cycle. My sleep cycle then becomes slightly disturbed. By Saturday, I have a sleep debt. I sleep a little longer, and the sleep is less restful. I also have more tired periods during the day that follows.

Chart your sleep week by week to gauge your sleep time. Once you have a clear picture of your current sleep pattern, you can begin to experiment. Try adjusting the time you start to sleep and the time you wake up. The optimum balance of sleep time and wake time occurs when you feel rested and refreshed for most of the day (when most of the daytime hours on your sleep chart are coded as H).

After experimenting for awhile, you should have a good picture of how much sleep you need. This key piece of information tells you one of the key steps to natural balance for your brain and your body. The amount of sleep you need becomes your first rule for living. Your program of sleep balance starts with this first natural rule for sleep balance:

Rule #1: Get the Right Amount of Healthy Sleep

Whenever your life feels out of balance, you can begin to restore balance by making sure that you sleep the right amount of time each day. By doing so, you are making sure that your brain and body are rested, that your energy stores are renewed, that you are physically ready for the challenges of life.

There are times in life when it is difficult to get the right amount of sleep. For me, that has happened three times: when I was an intern, training to be a doctor, and when my two children were infants. At those times, understanding my own natural rules for sleep really helped. Knowing that I need seven hours of sleep helped me accept the facts and to plan some solutions. I knew that days after I had slept less, for instance, when I was up at night with my son or daughter, or awake all night caring for a person who was deathly ill in the intensive care unit, on those days following inadequate sleep, I would be tired, a little grumpy and less alert. Understanding my sleep needs helped me to accept that my brain wouldn't work after missing sleep.

Understanding my sleep rules also helped me plan. If I could, I would find time for naps to catch up. If I knew that there was an activity that required me to be mentally sharp, I tried to plan a brief nap just before it. And knowing that I had a sleep deficit, I tried to avoid evening activities the night after I lost out on sleep.

These times happen to everyone. In today's world, common reasons for not being able to get enough sleep include:

- a new baby
- travel, especially across time zones
- exams at school
- deadlines at work
- taking care of an ill family member

- living in a noisy place
- working at night.

But you can help yourself in these circumstances. Start by developing a sleep chart. Understand your personal need for sleep. Then you can take some steps to help yourself adapt to a period of time when life prevents you from sleeping the right amount. Here are some ideas.

- Sleep the right number of hours: Using your sleep chart, determine the optimum length of sleep for your healthy functioning. Then try to get that amount of sleep every twenty-four hours. It is best, of course, if your sleep is uninterrupted. But there is strong evidence that getting the right amount of sleep, even if it is broken up into smaller segments, is helpful. Let's say you are awakened every night by your child's two o'clock feeding. You lose two hours of sleep as a result. It may help you to take a nap in the afternoon, to catch up on the needed sleep. One tip: It does not help to lengthen your sleep, by sleeping late into the morning. This can actually make matters worse. A nap later in the day is more helpful.
- Use "catnaps" to sharpen your mental function: Brief "catnaps"—naps that last up to fifteen minutes—can, by changing the physical state of your nervous system, reset the energy connections of your mind. If you have not been able to get enough sleep, and if you have a demanding task, such as a meeting or an exam, then a brief catnap can sharpen your mind,

renewing your mental energy, at least for a time.

- Plan your activities: Understand that you will not be sharp if you have not had enough sleep. Try to plan so that you have less mentally demanding tasks on days when you have not had enough sleep. Try to avoid dangerous activities like driving a car long distances or operating construction equipment when you have not had enough sleep.

- Find someone to help you so you can get some sleep: If you are taking care of an infant, make sure that you and your spouse share the night duties. Working nights? Find someone to help you with daytime chores so you can get enough sleep. Taking care of an ill family member? Make sure that all members of the family share the burden of care. If you can, try to hire some help to provide overnight coverage. Traveling for work? Make sure that someone from the local office helps you out as your body works to recover lost sleep.

Understand your need for sleep. Understand how much sleep your body and mind need for healthy functioning. Once you understand this natural rule, unique to you, then you can take steps to live in balance. And if the flow of your life prevents you from getting enough sleep, use your knowledge of this natural rule to help you to take steps, to adjust your life to minimize the impact of being unable to sleep the right amount. Sometimes, in our twenty-four hour society, that is the best thing you can do.

Better Sleep Through Chemicals?

Michael came to see me for consultation because he was depressed. As it turned out, Michael had another problem—a severe problem with sleep balance. His sleep problem was so bad, Michael was at risk of losing his job and his marriage.

Blessed with native intelligence, Michael had always performed at a high level. He breezed through college and through business school. After business school, he was offered a job with a prestigious Boston bank.

A good athlete, Michael complemented his studies with sports and exercise. He played baseball in college on a scholarship. In business school, he found time to work out every day.

Soon after he finished business school, he married. Michael and Sue had wonderful start to life, successful careers and a loving relationship.

The first sign of trouble for Michael had to do with disagreements he and Sue had about the hours Michael worked at the bank. As a junior executive at the bank, Michael worked long hours, frequently staying until late at night and on weekends. For good reason, Sue became more and more upset with Michael. She missed him. He was so pressed for time that he stopped his morning workout.

To be able to spend any time at all with Sue, Michael would come home from work, have dinner with Sue, relaxing with her for an hour or two. Later, after she had gone to bed, Michael stayed up to work. On the weekends, he caught up on sleep.

Although he started to feel tired much of the time, this schedule seemed like the best that he could do. It worked for Michael and Sue until Michael's father died. It was sudden.

Michael's dad was only sixty-three. Out of the blue, a massive heart attack took his life.

Michael and his dad had always been close. He had been a guiding influence for Michael; he always felt that he could turn to his dad for advice. So when his father died suddenly, it hit Michael hard. He grieved. He couldn't sleep. He felt exhausted all of the time. Sudden waves of sadness washed over him at unpredictable times. Work became overwhelming.

Concerned for Michael, Sue encouraged Michael to talk with his doctor. He did. His doctor diagnosed Michael with depression. He prescribed an antidepressant for him.

Unfortunately, since Michael's sleep was already out of balance from long hours at work and from grief, the antidepressant had the unintended effect of making Michael's sleep balance worse. The medication made him more sleepy and tired. Confused by this, thinking it was a sign that Michael's depression was worsening, his doctor gradually increased the dose of medication, inadvertently worsening Michael's problem.

When he came to see me, Michael was sleeping fourteen to sixteen hours per day. Yet despite this, he was tired all of the time. He was prone to falling asleep at any time of the day. He could not concentrate. His thinking was muddled. Convinced that work contributed to his depression, Michael took a leave of absence from his job. Originally he asked for two weeks, but the weeks turned into months and he was still no better. His boss at the bank threatened to fire him.

Each day Michael slept until noon. Then he would wake up, eat and watch television. Unable to get himself off the couch, Michael napped in the afternoon. He would wake up again when Sue came home from work. After dinner, Sue and

Michael would watch television together. Michael would begin to feel more alert in the evening. He would at least try to do some reading, but unable to keep his thoughts from ruminating about work, about his dad and about the fact that he felt like a failure, Michael found that he could not read or work. Then, when he tried to go to bed, he couldn't fall asleep. Every night, this convinced him that he needed the antidepressant. He would take the medicine and after lying awake in bed for another two hours he would fall asleep—only to repeat the cycle the next day.

Sue was becoming frustrated with Michael. He slept all of the time. Michael demonstrated no interest in her, his passion was gone. Thinking that he no longer loved her, and that he would not help himself, Sue began to talk with Michael about ending their marriage.

What happened to Michael? The circumstances of his life caused him to lose balance—his job, his new marriage, the death of his father, all contributed. Then the natural grief he suffered at the death of his father was labeled "depression." A medication was prescribed for this "depression." But the medicine made Michael worse by completely upsetting the natural balance of his sleep.

What did Michael need? Here is what worked for him. We gradually reduced and stopped the medication. This cleared up the medication-induced sleepiness. Michael started to exercise again, in the morning. He returned to work, while cutting back on his hours. Michael met with a therapist, to deal with the grief he still felt over his father's death and to provide a confiding relationship, of the kind that he had with his father. Over a six-month period, Michael's sleep balance returned to normal.

The fact that we have chemicals and medications which interfere with sleep is another indicator of the way in which our modern inventions—in this case, the thousands of medications and chemicals that have been created to treat illness and solve our problems in life—can subtly unbalance life. Michael's story illustrates the way in which you can lose your sleep balance and the balance in your life when you ingest modern chemicals—medications usually—that interfere with naturally balanced sleep.

It is quite a problem. Sleeping medications are the most commonly prescribed medications in this country. Over-the-counter cold medicines all contain chemicals that can interfere with sleep. Diet remedies like Dexatrim contain chemicals that interfere with your natural sleep balance. Performance enhancers, used by athletes to boost athletic performance, contain chemicals that interfere with sleep balance. Many prescription medications, such as antidepressants, high blood pressure medications, anti-anxiety medications, asthma medications, steroids and stimulant medications used for attention problems and narcolepsy, though important medications, can destroy the natural balance of your sleep.

Caffeine is a stimulant that can block naturally balanced sleep. The fact that caffeine is everywhere is a result of the problems with sleep balance that are endemic to our culture. That is why Starbucks, the chain of gourmet coffee shops, is one of the fastest-growing companies in the country. Caffeine shows up in a surprising number of substances: sometimes as a naturally occurring substance, and sometimes by design of the manufacturer. Caffeine, of course, is in all types of coffee and tea. High levels of caffeine are in most soft drinks such as Coke, Pepsi and Mountain Dew. Even orange soda contains high levels of caffeine! There is caffeine in chocolate. Caffeine is the active compound in over-the-counter medicines, used to keep you awake. Caffeine is in many pain pills, like Excedrin. Caffeine is in headache preparations. Once you start to read labels, you will see that caffeine is everywhere.

For our purposes, chemicals that affect sleep balance can be divided into two broad classes: those that enhance wakefulness and those that enhance sleepiness. In medical jargon, wakefulness-inducing chemicals are called stimulants. Sleep-inducing chemicals are called sedatives.

Chemicals That Make You Wake Up

Stimulants work by enhancing the activity of your wake cells, in the brain stem. Chemically, this happens in a variety of ways. Stimulants like methylphenidate work by stimulating the wake cells in the brain stem. Other stimulants, like caffeine, work by mimicking the chemical effect of your awake cells in your higher brain centers. The end result is that your higher brain centers are stimulated into action.

When you ingest a stimulant you become more alert, more energetic and more mentally active. This can feel good.

Problems occur when you habitually use a stimulant chemical to block the onset of sleep. Or, more commonly, when inadvertently the stimulant chemical interferes with restful sleep because the stimulant is still active in your bloodstream and in your brain at a time of day when you should be sleeping. This is what occurs when you drink coffee or some other caffeine-containing beverage in the afternoon or evening. It is a common problem when treating asthma with medicines like albuterol. It is a common problem when using stimulants like methylphenidate to treat an attention problem.

Sometimes, you must use a chemical (usually a prescription medication) that has a stimulant effect on your brain. If this is the case, then the best thing to do is to try and limit the use of the stimulant to early in the day. Then use some of the tools listed in the section on sleep structure, to help you to overcome the effects of the stimulant. In other words, if you must use a medication that is a stimulant, you will need to be certain to use the rules for sleep structure to help your brain know when to sleep and when to wake up.

Chemicals That Make You Sleepy

Sedatives or chemicals that make you sleepy work by mimicking the effects of your sleep cells. Sedatives actually shut off or inhibit the activity of the nerve cells in your neocortex. This makes you fall asleep. Sometime this is desirable; when you are having trouble falling asleep this can be helpful. Other times, it can be a nuisance; when you are taking a medication for other reasons, the fact that the medicine makes you sleep can be a problem.

When it comes to the balance of sleep and wakefulness, the real difficulty arises when sedative medications "trick" your nervous system into thinking that it is time for sleep, when the natural rhythm of your sleep clock may be telling you to wake up. For example, if you were to stay up all night to finish a project, then at 4 o'clock in the morning take a sedative to get you to sleep, you would be inadvertently desynchronizing your sleep clock. The most common way that this happens is when you take a sleep medication late at night to overcome a problem falling asleep. Then, the sleep medication causes you to sleep late into the morning. When you miss your usual wakeup time, when you miss exposure to morning light and morning activity, your sleep clock loses its rhythm. Then the next night, you have *more* trouble falling asleep! This is what happened to Michael. The antidepressant he was taking caused him to oversleep, and in doing so, it totally upset the natural cycle and structure of his sleep.

To complicate matters, many medications make you sleepy, when you are taking them for another purpose entirely. Here is a partial list of medications that can make you sleepy and by doing so, unbalance your sleep cycle.

- allergy medicines like Benadryl
- most cold medications like Contac
- high blood pressure medications like Inderal
- antidepressants like Pamelor, Remeron and Serzone
- pain medications like Percocet and Percodan
- herbal anxiety preparations like Kava kava
- anti-anxiety medications like Xanax and Klonopin
- anti-seizure medications like Dilantin
- reproductive hormones like progesterone

It is tempting to think that advances in modern

technologies are all related to machines. The truth of the matter is that machines and gadgets are only one part of the story. Advances in medicine and advances in chemistry have a more profound effect on how we live than almost any other scientific advance. You only have to think of the countless lives that have been saved by antibiotics to understand. Or the abundance of food on our tables, made possible by chemical fertilizers and pesticides. Although advances in medicine and chemistry do not have as obvious an impact as something like the automobile, the impact is still every bit as profound.

Modern medications can restore a healthy balance to life. Modern chemicals can make life more abundant. But the unintended consequences of the use of modern medicines can be that you lose balance. And this effect is at its worst when it comes to the impact of medications and chemicals on your sleep.

Many medications, many chemicals, can destroy the natural rhythm of your sleep cycle, causing you to oversleep or undersleep. Even though you may be using the medicine for a perfectly good reason—taking a medicine to control your blood pressure, or to treat your depression are good examples—the unintended effect, as it was for Michael, is that you lose your natural sleep balance.

Of course, using medications can save your life. Using medications can certainly help you feel better. The question we must face is: "How can you maintain a natural sleep balance, how can you preserve a healthy balance of energy and thought, when you must use a medication for your health?"

There is an answer. The answer lies in the balance

between the lower centers of your brain and the higher centers of your brain. The answer to this modern dilemma is to understand how to live in balance, within the helpful structure of the natural rules that set your sleep cycle. Learn to use your mind; understand the key variables that control your sleep clock; set your life to work in a harmonious rhythm—the natural cycling of your sleep clock.

For sleep is balanced in the same way as the other functions of your mind, through a harmonious linkage of the lower centers of your brain and the higher centers of your brain. Sleep is balanced when the cycling of your sleep clock works in harmony with your personal needs. That is balance.

How Is Sleep Balanced?

At the deepest level of your brain, in the brain stem, sleep is automatically balanced by the reciprocal action of two sets of nerve cells. Your awake cells stimulate all of your brain into an alert and wakeful state. After a time, your sleep cells automatically start to work, shutting off your awake cells so that you sleep.

There is an internal rhythm to the cycling of your sleep-center nerve cells. A full cycle lasts about twenty-five hours. If you lived in a cave, isolated from external cues about day and night, your daily cycle of waking and sleeping would run free, gradually lengthening until it reached the natural intrinsic rhythmicity of the cells in your sleep centers, running through a full cycle of sleep and wakefulness every twenty-five to twenty-eight hours. Researchers have actually proven this by living in a cave for long periods of time. If this occurred, your sleep cycle would be described as "running free."

If your sleep cycle ran free, then your daily cycle of sleep and rest would not match the daily needs of your life. You would be sleeping when you should be awake and you would be awake when it is time to sleep. It is even more complicated than this. Because your intrinsic sleep rhythm never stops moving forward, if your sleep cycle were to run free, the time that sleep starts and the time that you wake up would shift slightly later with each sleep cycle. So if your sleep cycle ran free, your sleep time and your wake time would change every day, in a gradually lengthening cycle.

Now, imagine a free-running sleep cycle in the life of our prehistoric ancestors. A free-running cycle with unpredictable periods of sleep and wakefulness, out of synch with the natural cycles of day and night, would not be compatible with life. It would interfere with hunting and gathering food. It would interfere with caring for family. It would expose you to life-threatening risks from predators and from aggression by marauding gangs of aggressive humans. It would expose you to the elements in a dangerous way.

Common sense tells you that this sequence of events did not happen. Nature, in its wisdom, would not create a sleep cycle that was dangerous to you. What correction was made? The correction was balance. A natural and harmonious balance developed that corrected for this sleep-programming flaw. The human brain developed in such a way that you reset your internal sleep clock and your sleep centers every day by structure you provide from cues natural to your environment.

Sleep researchers call this process *entrainment*. Every day, you are surrounded by a world of cues that tell you and your sleep centers, when to be awake and when to sleep. From obvious cues like an alarm clock and the onset of night, to more subtle cues like temperature, activity patterns and diet, your sleep centers are set, like a clock, into a sleep cycle that matches your environment.

Nature has made your sleep cycle exquisitely sensitive to environmental cues and to the circumstances in your life. As you structure your day-to-day life to meet your needs and to match your preferences, your body gathers information about the environment. This information is channeled through an important processing center called the hypothalamus. A signal is sent to your sleep centers that adjusts your sleep clock to the needs of your life.

Here are some of the cues that set, or entrain, your sleep clock:

environmental cue	effect on the sleep clock
bright morning light	earlier wake time; earlier sleep time
morning darkness	later wake time
alerting sounds in the morning	earlier wake time

alerting sounds at night	later sleep time
afternoon exercise	earlier sleep time; earlier wake time
evening milk or carbohydrate meal	earlier sleep time
dieting or decreased caloric intake	earlier wake time
warm room	earlier wake time
cool room	delayed wake time
mental stimulation in the morning	earlier wake time
mental stimulation at night	delayed sleep time; delayed wake time

In prehistoric times the human brain clock was efficiently adjusted to make sure that periods of wakefulness were timed to improve your chances of survival. You can see the natural logic of this system. Signals that cause your wake time to shift earlier result in more wakefulness during the day. Putting it another way, sunlight, the warmth of the day, strange or unpredictable noises, mental stimulation (like worry), and hunger signal your brain to wake up and to be prepared for action.

Conversely, darkness in the morning, cool temperatures and a quiet environment are a signal to snuggle into the blankets and sleep for longer periods. These cues go along with the seasonal change in day length. As the days become shorter and the nights longer, your brain senses this, telling you to sleep longer and later into the day.

In the same way, a carbohydrate meal tends to make you sleepy. Carbohydrates are turned directly into energy stores, like fat. The hormones that produce this change make you sleepy. This is like a hibernation response. Your brain senses that you are eating a lot of carbohydrates and interprets this as a message that it is time to start to hibernate.

Sleep and wakefulness are balanced naturally, when your sleep clock is set to cycle in harmony with your environment, in such a way that you have predictable, restful and effective sleep.

With everything that is possible today, in our twenty-four-hour-per-day, nonstop world, when you can do just about anything, just about anytime that you want to, the exquisite sensitivity of your sleep clock works against you. Why? Because your brain was created to adjust your sleep cycle, your sleep clock, to changes in your life circumstances and to changes in your environment. And, we modern humans change everything about our environment and circumstances all the time. We fly across time zones changing the length of the day and the timing of sunrise. We travel from cold climates to warm climates and from warm climates to cold climates. We can eat any type of meal whenever we want. We can stay up late at night, turned on by the mental stimulation of television and the Internet. We can work, shop, socialize or study any time of the day or night. We can change any of this at any time.

What happens to sleep? It becomes unbalanced by life.

Your sleep clock never sets into a predictable rhythm, or it sets itself into an unhealthy rhythm. When your sleep clock is not functioning in a natural, healthy balance with your life, then you lose your sleep balance. Your sleep becomes unstructured, erratic, inefficient and unrestful. When your sleep is out of balance, you will not have the benefit of the natural renewal and energy restoration that only comes from naturally balanced sleep. If your sleep is out of balance long enough, then you will not feel well; you will not perform well; you will not be at your best.

The modern paradox is that all of the possibility of modern life unbalances your sleep clock and prevents you from being physically able to get as much from life as you might want. The limitless possibilities of modern life interfere with the natural balance of your sleep cycle, preventing you from being able to take advantage of all that modern life has to offer. The biologic fact is that your sleep clock must operate in a natural balance with your life; you must get efficient, well-timed and restful sleep or you will not be able to function at your best. And if your sleep imbalance becomes extreme, it can literally make you sick.

Since, in our Western culture, we long ago decided that body and mind are unconnected, it never occurs to us that this is a problem. In our culture, because we can be so mentally stimulated all of the time, our view of sleep has changed. Because we value hard work, intelligence, mental stimulation and information, we have lost sight of the fact that sleep is essential to a healthy life. Instead, we view the need to sleep as a type of personal failure. In our society, we give in to sleep as though finally deciding to sleep were an admission of laziness or failure.

This contrasts with the natural facts: to be healthy, you *must* sleep the right amount for you and you *must* sleep in a way that is right for you. To put this in perspective consider this phrase, "You must breathe." It seems a little silly since we all accept that a regular breathing cycle is necessary for life. Now consider this phrase, "You must sleep." To most people, the phrase "You must sleep" just does not carry the weight of the phrase "You must breathe." Our beliefs and our culture tell us that sleeping is not as essential to life as breathing is, that we can control our sleep, that we need not *give in* to sleep. Can you imagine telling anyone that you don't need to *give in* to breathing? It would be absurd. Well, it is just as absurd to imagine that you need not *give in* to sleep. To your body, and especially to your brain, naturally balanced sleep is as essential to health as breathing.

Instead of thinking that sleep interferes with work or socializing, the healthy and balanced view is to learn how to use the power of your thinking mind in harmony with the energy-generating process of your sleep cycle. You can use all that you know about yourself, all that you know about the circumstances of your life, and all that you know about the regulation of your sleep cycle to produce a healthy balance of sleep and wakefulness. When you live in balance you can sleep and when you sleep, you can live in balance.

Here is a story about Tom. It is a story about the way that Tom lost the balance in his sleep. It is a story about regaining balance in difficult circumstances.

Pulling All-Nighters
Caught Up with Him

Tom was in my office to talk with me about some difficulty he was having at school.

"I just can't focus in class," he said. Tom had come to see me because he was tired all of the time, and because he was not getting the grades in college that he expected.

"I should be doing better. But my mind wanders in class. When I try to do the reading . . . forget about it! I read and reread the same page and nothing sinks in."

It was ten o'clock in the morning when Tom consulted me. A good-looking man, with sandy blond hair and an easy smile, Tom's green eyes shine with intelligence. But that morning, he looked tired. He was unshaven, dressed in a wrinkled yellow and green warm-up suit. It was the middle of the morning, a bright and clear April day. Yet he looked as though he was ready to crawl into bed or to collapse on the couch.

An intelligent and hard-working man, Tom had some ambitious goals.

"I plan to finish college in three years by going full time. The university has an evening program, where you can get full-time credits. I work nights as a security guard at the medical center to earn a living."

"When do you study?" I asked.

"I can study on my breaks at work, if I can stay awake. I do most of my studying when I get home from work, in the morning," he replied.

"When do classes start?" I asked. It was beginning to sound like there wasn't enough time for Tom to do everything.

"At five o'clock."

"And when do you sleep?" I asked. Tom glanced out the window and paused. This is something that always happens when I ask people about sleep. The long pause, indicating that we are about to discuss a sensitive topic.

"I get enough sleep," Tom responded quickly, defensively. He reacted as though I had asked him if he was stealing from the church collection plate. "On the weekends, I sleep in as much as twelve hours."

"Can you tell me what time you go to sleep and what time you wake up?" I asked him.

"I get to bed around eleven and sleep until 2:30." He paused again and tried to avoid my gaze.

"When do you socialize and when do you have time for exercise?"

"I don't," Tom replied. "I had to give those things up. I don't have the time," he answered. "The funny thing is, I don't miss them either. It's like I've lost interest in them."

"Do you need to pull all-nighters?" I asked.

"Not at first I didn't. But as the semester has gone on, I've had to do two or three all-nighters per week to get all of the work done. But I catch up on my sleep on the weekends. If I could just focus better I wouldn't have to skip so much sleep. I'm working hard, probably twice as hard as other people in my class. But the material just won't stick. I'm afraid I'm too stupid for college. So I figure if I want to go to college, I've got to cut back on sleep and work harder. I was hoping that you could help me out."

"What did you have in mind, Tom?"

"Well, I'm tired all of the time. And I doze off while I'm studying. I was hoping you could prescribe something to help me stay awake when I need to study," Tom replied, wearing a hopeful expression.

"Before I do that, Tom, I need to know how your health is, in general."

"That's easy. I just had a checkup. I've been breaking out in sweats when I study. And I've had such a hard time remembering, I thought maybe I was sick. But I'm okay. My primary-care doc told me that I had a virus, and that my blood pressure was a little high, but other than that I'm in great shape."

Tom's sleep cycle was out of synch with his life. He had lost a healthy sleep balance, and it was beginning to affect his health. Totally absorbed in his goal of finishing college, Tom became driven by work and by school. And as he did, Tom lost the structure of his sleep.

"To be truthful, I sleep when I can. Sometimes I sleep in the afternoon. Sometimes I catch a few winks at work. Sometimes, if I have things to do, I don't sleep at all."

I was able to convince Tom that he might be more alert and that he might feel better if we could make some simple changes in his sleep schedule. He agreed, at least as an experiment, to give it a try.

Our first step was to set a routine sleep time and a routine wake time. Tom got home from work at 8:00 A.M. With an hour to relax, 9:00 A.M. seemed to be a reasonable sleep time. Since Tom felt he needed seven hours of sleep, we set 4:00 P.M. as his wake time. Getting seven hours of sleep was Tom's first rule of sleep balance.

To help to strengthen his sleep cycle, I had Tom buy a sun-box, to provide him with bright light. He sat in front of the light from 3:30 to 4:00 while he ate his breakfast.

To help his sleep, Tom bought an air-conditioner, room-darkening blinds and white noise machine.

With these changes, Tom slept more soundly. He felt more alert when he was working. Since he had long breaks at work, between the times he made his night rounds, Tom was able to catch up on his studying. His supervisors were okay with this, as long as he was awake and at his post.

I instructed Tom to stay with this sleep schedule on weekends, too. Trying to shift back to a regular day-night schedule on weekends was destabilizing his sleep cycle. Since he wasn't working, Tom then had extra time, during the hours that were his normal work hours, to catch up on his studying.

"I'm sleeping better, Doc, but I don't have enough time to catch up on errands," Tom told me.

To save money, Tom was living at home with his parents. I suggested that he talk with them, to see if they could help.

"My dad said he would be glad to do a few things for me. He figured I was working so hard to pay my tuition bill, that it was the least he could do to help out."

By following a few natural rules, Tom was able to establish some balance. He felt better and his grades were improving. Tom was convinced.

"I took it a step further. I found a way to get some exercise at work. There is a gym at the medical center. I use it on my last break. You know, a quick workout. It helps me to get to sleep faster when I get home."

Here are the natural rules that Tom followed to establish a healthy sleep balance.

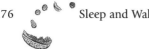

> ### Tom's Rules for Sleep Balance
>
> 1. *Try to get seven hours of sleep per day.*
> 2. *Go to sleep at 9:00 A.M. and wake up at 4:00 P.M. every day. Don't shift on weekends.*
> 3. *Use bright light to strengthen his sleep cycle.*
> 4. *Create a healthy sleep environment.*
> 5. *Get help from his dad.*

Feeling better, more energetic and thinking more clearly, Tom was convinced. He used his rules for sleep balance to keep up with his demanding schedule. And he succeeded. He reached his goals while staying in a healthy balance.

How Can You Structure and Balance Sleep?

Problems with sleep structure are a silent epidemic. In all segments of society, the demands of a twenty-four hour-per-day culture upset the structure of sleep. From high school students staying awake until 3:00 A.M. to use the Internet, to high-tech engineers working all night on the latest software products, to mothers up at night caring for sick children, paying bills, trying to keep the house clean because there is no time during the day.

The way that you sleep can be as important as how much sleep you get. The timing and structure of your day and of your sleep can determine how well-balanced your sleep clock really is. In order to feel your best; in order to be at your best, your sleep clock must function in a rhythmic balance with your personal preferences and with your personal needs.

The challenge that you face is the excitement and the abundance of modern life. There are so many factors in our culture interfering with the structure of our sleep that it takes an active and sustained effort to set our sleep clocks into a naturally balanced rhythm.

Consider these everyday matters. Each can upset the balance of your sleep clock: air travel across time zones (jet lag), artificial lighting, night work, late-night television, the Internet, daylight savings time, late-night phone calling (from coast to coast), lack of exercise, sleeping late into the morning, late-night restaurants, twenty-four-hour-per-day shopping, to name just a few.

All of these activities interfere with the natural set of your sleep clock. All of these activities keep your sleep cycle from becoming *entrained* by the natural cycle of day and night. All of these modern-day activities prevent you from living in natural balance. Before you know it, like Tom, your sleep becomes unstructured and you begin to suffer the problems that go along with not getting enough restful sleep. To make matters worse, when your sleep cycle begins to run free, your pattern of sleep can become out of synch with the rest of life. The most common pattern is to stay awake much of the night, finally falling asleep at 3:00 or 4:00 A.M., causing your wake time to be delayed until 10:00 or 11:00 A.M.

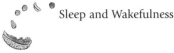

Lack of sleep structure often leads to problems with prescription medications and with alcohol. Since your sleep clock runs free, it tells you to sleep at inconvenient times. Conversely, when you finally have time to sleep, your sleep clock can be telling you to stay awake. In our society, the solution to this problem is to chemically induce sleep with medications and with alcohol. This can lead to addiction to the sleep medicine. Your body quickly becomes dependent on the prescription medication to induce sleep. Then, you must have it.

Alcohol presents even more of a problem. It is readily available, so the temptation can be great to reach for a drink as a solution for sleeplessness. But, while alcohol is a mild sedative—it makes you sleepy an hour or so after you have a drink—alcohol is toxic to sleep. It completely disrupts the process of restful sleep. It completely disrupts the functioning of your sleep clock. If you use alcohol to help you sleep, your brain quickly becomes addicted to alcohol. The sleep-disrupting effects of alcohol backfire on you, so that you then have to have a drink to get to sleep. This can lead to serious alcohol troubles and alcoholism.

To find out if you have a problem with the structure and timing of your sleep, answer these questions.

Do You Have Trouble with the Structure of Your Sleep?

1. Do you wake up at a different time each day?   yes   no
2. Do you get to sleep at a different time each night?   yes   no
3. Do you take naps so that you can stay up later at night?   yes   no

4. If you do nap, do you then have
   trouble falling asleep at bedtime?   yes   no
5. Do you sleep late on weekends and
   holidays to catch up?   yes   no
6. Do you stay up late to work, read, watch
   TV, use the computer, to eat and socialize
   or to talk on the phone?   yes   no
7. Do you watch TV in bed and then have
   trouble falling asleep?   yes   no
8. Do you stay up all night to
   meet deadlines?   yes   no
9. Do you have trouble quieting your mind
   when you try to sleep?   yes   no
10. Do you travel across time zones
    at least once a week?   yes   no
11. Do you take a sleeping pill or drink
    alcohol to help you to get to sleep?   yes   no

Score_____

If you answered yes to three or more of these questions, the problem you have with the balance of sleep and wakefulness, may be caused by a problem of sleep structure.

There is quite a lot you can do about this type of problem. Remember, earlier in this chapter we reviewed the way in which your sleep clock and your sleep cycle is set by the circumstances of your life. Well, that is the key to structuring your sleep. You can use these natural sleep cues to create a prescription of balance for your sleep structure. Understand your natural sleep cues; understand that your sleep cues are your natural rules for sleep balance; learn to structure your sleep and to reset your sleep clock.

As you read through this section, reflect on how these rules of sleep structure can have an impact on your life. Reflect on these questions. Which of the rules make sense for you? Which rules are practical for you? Which rules for living might you want to try? Every rule is not for every person. You may want to pick two or three and try them. Experiment a bit. Use your sleep chart to see which of the sleep structure rules have the most beneficial impact on your sleep cycle. Then, when you determine which of the rules work best for you, make them a regular part of your program of balance.

Rule #1: Set a Routine Time to Wake Up and Get Out of Bed—Then Stick to It

The time that you wake up and get out of bed sends a powerful signal to your sleep clock. Your wake-up time sets your sleep-cycle clock ticking. When you wake up at the same time every day, you are training your sleep clock to function predictably. By doing this, your circadian rhythm will be set so that you are alert early in the day, and you are at your sleepiest about sixteen hours later. You may need help with this. A reliable alarm clock can be useful. Probably the best assistance you can get is from another person who awakens you at the prescribed time. Remember, it is not enough to simply wake up, you must also get out of bed and become active.

Rule #2: Expose Yourself to Bright Light When You Wake Up

Bright light when you wake up also sets your sleep clock. The best way to get bright light is to go outside for a walk. If that is not possible, then use a bright light for at least thirty minutes in the morning. You will need a very bright light, that provides at least 2,500 lux of light intensity. Some people put the bright light on the countertop, sitting in front of it while having coffee and reading the morning paper.*

Rule #3: Exercise in the Afternoon

Late-afternoon exercise also sets your sleep clock and triggers the onset of sleep. Any exercise will do. One way (among many ways) that exercise works is by raising your heart rate and your body temperature. The abrupt cooling after exercise works to set your sleep clock. For this to be effective, the exercise should not be closer than three hours to bedtime.

Rule #4: Organize Your Activity So That Mentally Stimulating Activity Occurs Early in the Day, Soon After You Wake Up

Mental stimulation is another signal to set your sleep clock. It works by helping your awake cells to function better. Mental stimulation sends the same type of chemical message to your brain as your wake cells do. And when you enhance the function of your wake cells early in the day, you also trigger the function of your sleep cells about sixteen hours later.

---

*A good place to buy a bright light is Northern Lights Technologies. They can be reached at 1-800-263-0066.

Rule #5: Eat Regularly Timed Meals; Avoid Snacking at Night

Regular meals also work to set your sleep clock. If you are hungry or not eating regularly, it can have the opposite effect, interfering with restful sleep and upsetting the natural rhythm of your sleep clock. The only exception to this is that milk or a *light* snack of carbohydrates (like bread, pasta or crackers) can help trigger the onset of sleep.

Rule #6: Create a Sleep-Inducing Atmosphere Two Hours Before Your Planned Sleep Time

A sleep-inducing atmosphere is one that enhances the function of your sleep cells. Soft lighting, quiet rhythmic activity (like knitting) and physical relaxation all help your sleep cells to function better and, by extension, to set your sleep clock. You can enhance this effect by learning to use a relaxation technique, such as meditation or progressive relaxation, in the pre-sleep time. Avoid any activity that is mentally or emotionally stimulating, such as television watching, reading mystery novels or surfing the Internet.

Rule #7: Make Sure That the Place You Sleep Helps You to Sleep

The ideal sleep environment is a dark, quiet, cool room with a physically comfortable bed (or sleeping surface). Each of these characteristics enhances the function of your sleep cells, thereby deepening sleep. When you deepen sleep, you enhance the function of your sleep clock.

Conversely a noisy, warm, bright place where you are physically uncomfortable (like in an airplane!) sends wake-up messages to your brain, prompting your wake cells to become active. This will wake you up and upset the natural balance of your sleep clock.

Rule #8: Take a Hot Bath in the Evening

Like exercise, a hot bath sends a powerful signal that triggers your sleep cells into action. It seems to work in the same way: a rise in body temperature while in your bath, followed by an abrupt cooling after the bath, sends a message for your sleep cells to go to work. A hot bath can be a useful tool to help you get to sleep when you want and to help you to reset your sleep clock into a healthy balance.

Rule #9: Avoid Alcohol

Alcohol produces a double whammy of sleep disruption. Drinking alcohol can make you sleepy and cause you to fall asleep at a time that is out of synch with your sleep cycle. The more difficult problem is that as the alcohol leaves your system, it wakes you up. As little as two ounces of alcohol any time after three o'clock in the afternoon can have this effect. The regular use of alcohol frequently leads to sleep problems. A particular problem happens when you take a drink as a way of inducing sleep. In this circumstance, the cure (the nightcap) worsens the condition, causing you to drink more. So if your sleep is out of balance, if you have trouble structuring your sleep, stop drinking alcohol.

Sleep and Wakefulness Self-Test

Take this test to see if you are out of balance. If you answered yes to three or more questions, then you may have a problem with the balance of sleep and wakefulness. To improve your balance, try to incorporate the rules in this chapter as well as the tips to follow.

1. Do you often feel that no matter what you do, you cannot get enough sleep?　　yes　　no
2. Do you lie in bed awake, unable to fall asleep, causing you to oversleep in the morning?　　yes　　no
3. Do you take a sleeping pill or drink alcohol to help you to get to sleep?　　yes　　no
4. Do you wake up at a different time each day?　　yes　　no
5. Do you often stay up late to work, read, watch TV, use the computer, to eat and socialize, or to talk on the phone?　　yes　　no

Score _____

Tips to Balance Sleep and Wakefulness

1. Use a sleep chart like the ones on pages 251 and 252. Sleeping the right amount is fundamental to sleep balance. Fill out a sleep chart like the one displayed here to determine what is the right amount of sleep for you. Then, use the other natural rules for sleep and the tips listed here to help you to get the right amount of sleep.

   For each hour of the day put in a W, if you are awake, and an S if you are asleep. Then on the second line marked "state" put in the code for your energ state. If you are sleeping put in an R for restful sleep or a P for poor or restless sleep. For times that you are awake, code an H for a rested or high energy state, when you are feeling well. Code a T, for a low energy tired state. Then connect all of the W's, all of the S's, all of the H's and all of the T's.

After you keep this chart for a week you will have a picture of when you sleep, when you are awake and how you feel during those times.

2. Arrange for a wake-up call. Waking up at the same time every day sets your sleep into a healthy cycle. One way to make this happen is by asking someone to wake you up. It could be your spouse, your children, a sympathetic coworker, your parents or a friendly neighbor. Don't worry that you are imposing. Whoever you ask to wake you up will feel good about playing such a helpful role in your life.

3. Buy a recliner. If the circumstances of your life prevent you from getting enough sleep, taking catnaps, fifteen- minute naps in the middle of the day, can be a real life saver. Make sure you have a comfortable chair to sleep in . . . like a recliner. Try to avoid using your bed, as this might draw you into a longer nap which could upset your sleep cycle. It need not be a recliner that you sleep on. It could be a couch, the floor or a hammock. The essential elements are that you be comfortable but not in bed.

4. Put your bed in front of an east facing window. An east facing window will help you in several ways. You can open it, to cool your bedroom to a better

temperature for sleep. The morning sunlight from the rising sun will help to wake you on a predictable schedule. Exposure to morning light will strengthen your sleep cycle, making it easier to fall asleep the next night. And the brightness of the morning sun will help to jump-start your nervous system, so that you are alert and ready for the day.

5. Schedule meetings in the morning, read at night. Meetings can tax your brain, making it hard to fall asleep. Meeting with people can be a stimulating experience. If you need to meet with a group of people to discuss important matters, try to do so in the morning. The stimulation of the meeting will strengthen your natural cycle of morning alertness.

On the other hand, save your reading for night. As you move your eyes in the gentle back and forth rhythms of reading, it relaxes you. The subtle, physical calming that happens naturally when you read will work in synch with your sleep cycle, slowly moving you toward the relaxed state that precedes sleep.

6. Take the TV out of the bedroom. Television is a stimulating medium. Although watching television in bed is a luxury that many enjoy, it actually works against your natural cycle of sleep. Over time, if you watch enough television in bed, you can actually train your nervous system to become alert and stimulated whenever you lie down in your bed. If you enjoy relaxing in front of the tube, try doing it on the couch. Save your bedroom for sleeping.

7. Sleep on your stomach or your side, not on your

back. If you snore, sleeping on your back can interfere with restful sleep. As your muscles relax in sleep, the opening for your airway becomes smaller. This can block your breathing, cause snoring and interfere with restful sleep. In mild cases, simply sleeping on your stomach or your back prevents this problem.

8. Try a new bed. Your physical comfort is important to a healthy sleep balance. If you are physically uncomfortable, no matter what the reason, it can be difficult to get restful sleep. Think about how you feel when you sleep. If you are uncomfortable in some way, whether it is from snoring, from aches and pains in your joints or simply from an uncomfortable mattress, then it can be impossible to get a healthy and balanced sleep.

   One quick fix is to try a new bed, one that fits your unique body style and sleep habits. A host of sleep problems can simply disappear when you are sleeping in a bed that is right for you.

9. Drink coffee, but only in the morning. Must you avoid all caffeine? Certainly not. Coffee, tea and all types of caffeine, in moderation, taken in the morning can enhance your sleep cycle by strengthening the alerting process your brain needs early in the day. Problems arise when you use caffeine too late in the day. Then the residual effects of the caffeine can disturb your sleep. But if you like coffee, go ahead and indulge. Just do it before 11:00 A.M.

10. Try not to have alcohol two nights in a row.

Alcohol can put you to sleep but it also wakes you up. About three hours after your last drink, the alcohol quickly leaves your body. As it does, it wakes you up. Research has shown that as little as one drink in the evening causes you to have less restful sleep. One way to keep this from interfering with your sleep balance is by trying not to drink two nights in a row. This will help you to have healthier, more restful sleep on the night you abstain.

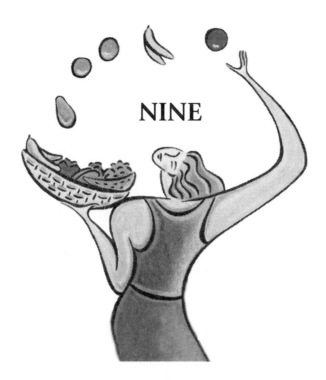

NINE

System 7:
Belief and Doubt

Without hoopla or fanfare, a patent clerk from Bern, Switzerland [Albert Einstein], had completely overturned the traditional notions of space and time and replaced them with a new conception whose properties fly in the face of everything we are familiar with from common experience.

Brian Greene, *The Elegant Universe*

It all comes together with belief: living in balance.

Sure, modern life is abundantly rich, stimulating, exciting and overwhelming. And there is no end of advice to help you to live right. In this book alone, you have now seen six different steps to balance with rules, tips and advice. How can you make sense of this? How can you put together a personal program that will lead to balance? How can you help yourself without falling into the trap of adding one more thing to learn, one more set of facts to comprehend, one more demand on you, on your time and on your life?

The answer is belief.

Your personal program of balance is woven together in a sensible pattern by adding belief to your life. Healthy, sustaining, confidence-boosting belief. Real belief, based on a firm understanding of who you are and how you operate best. A type of belief that guides your actions. For when your belief is strong, your life will move in smooth and flowing rhythms.

Why? Because that is how we are made. Your brain was created to function best when you are guided by strong beliefs. Like a conductor, skillfully blending the disparate musical elements that are the unique contribution of each musician, organizing, adding the right timing and emphasis, making sure that the music elements come together into the gorgeous unified sound of a symphony, belief guides, conducts and organizes the unique and important functional elements of your mind, into a unified, rhythmic, harmonious balance.

You can live in balance. It may be that only one element

of your life is out of balance. Not enough movement, perhaps. Or too much time alone. Or perhaps it is a matter of reintroducing yourself to your skills and abilities, to your identity as a person with a unique story. If so, then you will have already found your answer. But if your life is out of balance in a number of ways, if you are not sure how to make it all work, then you may find your answer in this chapter on belief. When you understand the central role of belief in establishing and maintaining your balance for life, then you will have a clear sense of how to live in balance.

The Illusion of Certainty and the Undermining of Belief

Let's start with an example from my own life that illustrates for you the way that modern life produces what I call "the illusion of certainty" and, by doing so, undermines the natural balance of belief.

It happened one day as I was driving home from work. At the time, Susan and I were living in Dayton, Ohio. Our home was in a pretty suburb, on a tree-lined street, up the hill from the Miami River and the main rail and highway corridor connecting Dayton to other parts of the industrial Midwest. It was the end of the day. After nine hours of working with people, talking on the phone and responding to pages, I was tired. But my mind was buzzing with energy; as I drove, sitting still, responding to the flow of traffic, I rolled thought after thought, memory after memory, over in my mind.

I had a twenty-mile drive from the hospital to my home in the suburbs; I had thirty minutes of sitting still while I drove and thought.

The radio played in the background. My thoughts gradually turned toward home, to my regular, after-work exercise, to a quiet meal and an evening to relax.

In the next instant, I was jolted to attention. With great drama, the news anchor described some "breaking news." A tank car carrying nitrogen phosphate had derailed in Carrolton. Firefighters on the scene reported that a deadly gas was leaking from the derailed tank car. Nearby homeowners were being evacuated.

The train yards in Carrolton were only a mile from my home. I became electrified with worry and fear: my home, my family, what would happen? My nervous system cried out in alarm. I wanted to do something to make it right, to keep my family and my home safe from this deadly gas. But, I was stuck in traffic on I-75. There was nothing I could do.

As I drove home slowly, in the rush hour traffic, the news reports grew steadily worse. Anyone living within five miles could be evacuated. The gas could ignite in a burst of flame. Any contact with the gas could cause severe breathing problems, even death. The radio announcer, in authoritative tones, reassured us, the listening audience, that we would be given all of the facts as they were made available.

Ready for the worst, I made my way home. As I turned the corner onto my street, to my surprise, I saw children playing on the street. The windows and doors of my home were open. Susan was inside, happily cooking dinner. I asked her if she knew about the deadly gas and the evacuation. No she responded, she hadn't heard a thing. Not a TV watcher or a radio listener, Susan had heard nothing.

Confused, I turned the TV on. Live pictures showed a tank car, with one wheel off the track, surrounded by men calmly surveying the scene. They were not wearing gas masks, they did not have chemical suits on. The leak, a tiny leak, had been sealed twenty minutes ago.

What had happened? The media had accurately reported some things. There was a derailment, there was a small leak. There was talk of evacuation and danger. But the leak was contained, the danger never materialized. It was easily and safely contained.

And I, alone in my car, listening to the news, became alarmed by the certainty that disaster was striking my home. Prior to hearing the breaking news, I felt calm. I felt safe. I believed my family and my home were safe. I believed that I would be able to conduct my nightly routine. I believed that I could relax after a long day at work. I believed that life was ordered, structured and predictable.

But the news, as I heard it, at least for the moment, shattered the comfort of my beliefs. The illusion of certainty put forth by the radio announcer, the certainty that disaster was striking my home, undermined the structure of my beliefs.

Now I am not going to say that this one episode put my life permanently out of balance. When I got home, I exercised as I always did. I had a quiet meal with my family. I relaxed with some reading. After a while, I was fine.

But this story portrays the way in which modern life undermined my natural beliefs in the safety, the security and rhythms of my life. At least for thirty minutes or so, the urgency of the "breaking news" I heard on the radio shattered my beliefs, and I was a nervous wreck.

Today, we are subject to "breaking news" all day long. We are surrounded by a parade of experts telling us what will or won't happen. We are told of power shortages, of weather disasters, of crime sprees and chemical spills with urgency, with immediacy and with drama.

It does not stop with disasters either. All day long you are flooded by images of experts telling you, with great certainty, about your life: how to exercise to be healthy, how to invest to be wealthy, where to shop for best values, what car to drive to be safe, the best ways to raise your children, how to work and how to play.

And then there are the pundits. On radio and TV, they critique and analyze everything from political speeches to who is the best teacher, from what medicines to buy to what exercise equipment works best. Not only do we have innumerable experts telling us, with great certainty, how to do everything, we have a chorus of pundits telling us which experts to believe.

The information age—television, radio, cell phones, faxes and e-mail—these miraculous technologies give you instant access to information. With great speed and urgency, you can gather facts and communicate with others. Instead of trusting your beliefs, you turn on the television, or pick up the telephone or log on to the Internet, in hopes that you can find out what is going on.

In hopes that you can figure out what to believe, what to do. The information age and the illusion of certainty have replaced personal belief with the false impression that you can gather enough facts, discover the accurate truth of a situation and then, based on these facts, make a decision about what to do.

It is a never-ending task.

As you have seen, it all comes at you in a constant flood, at great speed, with high drama, a sense of urgency and with an air of certainty. You are always given "the facts."

You react, of course, with your ancient brain, wired to respond to the reality of another age. Your mind seizes on the high drama; it quickly grasps the urgency; it interprets the new information in the way it was programmed to do—as a sign of danger. Because of the illusion of certainty, because of the speed, the drama, and the amount of factual data, your brain automatically begins to worry. The lower centers of your brain interpret all of this as a sign of danger. Confronted by a flood of important, new information, information presented powerfully, with an air of authority, challenged by a collection of new facts, presented to you as though you were hearing directly from a personal messenger, still breathless with the effort it took to reach you; your brain, naturally enough, interprets the message. Something new, something unforeseen, something dangerous, something that is a threat to your survival is looming on the horizon.

The natural belief in your own security, safety and the continuity of your day-to-day life comes under question. You begin to lose touch with these central beliefs. In the urgent moment of the information age, you doubt the very things that are most important to you. You live in a never-ending state of disbelief, worry and doubt.

Here is a list of factors that contribute to the under-mining of belief:

- you are presented with "factual information."
- the information is conveyed by experts.
- the story is given the aura of scientific certainty.
- the information is conveyed with bright colors, loud music and high drama.
- the information is presented as a sound bite, out of context.
- you are alone with the information.
- you are unable to react naturally.
- your attention is diverted from understanding the "factual information" by the next piece of informa-tion presented to you in this way.

This is happening all day, every day, in today's plugged-in world. Each day, the pace and urgency of modern life activates the alarm centers of your brain. Repeat this sce-nario day after day, hour after hour and eventually, your brain turns the constant alarm into a world view. Instead of living with the secure feeling of belief, instead of the peace that comes from understanding the natural order of life, instead of the confidence that comes from knowing how you fit, your brain turns the constant stimulation and alarm into worry, nervousness and doubt.

The problem is that our sped-up, digital-information

age technologies, combined with our love of high drama, convince us every day that our beliefs are unsound and that we can only know something by analyzing the facts. The truth of a situation is in the facts and how they come together.

Much of the time this is true. But for much of the time, it is not. It is just not possible to know everything all of the time. This god-like quality, the illusion of certainty, is unattainable.

In my story about the chemical spill, the radio announcer presented facts that sounded right. I believed my family and my home were in danger. It seemed possible to me that when I arrived home, I would find a hastily abandoned home, poisoned by a toxic gas. I doubted my beliefs about the safety of my family.

But the facts I heard, while accurate at the moment, were not the truth. The truth was not knowable at that moment. Had I never heard the radio report, my beliefs would have gone unchallenged. Or, had I been home if I did not work twenty miles away, if I did not have to spend thirty minutes alone in my car, my beliefs would not have been challenged. Or, if the news media, reporting in a way that is just not possible for the news media, had announced a different message, something like, "We have some preliminary and ambiguous news from Carrolton about a possible chemical spill, but don't worry, firefighters are on the scene and they appear to have the matter in control." My beliefs would not have been challenged and I would not have become as alarmed as I did. But as I lived my normal, modern life, I was a sitting duck for a crisis of belief.

On a moment-to-moment basis, that is how it happens. Challenged at every turn by facts and analysis, it becomes difficult to be certain what is actually going on. The antidote to this modern dilemma is belief. When you believe in yourself and in the wisdom of something larger than yourself, when you follow the practice of belief, the natural rules of belief, then the uncertainty dissolves and you begin to know what to do.

Here is a story about Kim, to show you how this works.

Never Comfortable Around Others

"I'm nervous all of the time," Kim explained. "I get nervous around people, in stores, even in church. It's even been hard for me to sit through Mass."

Since her children were grown, the youngest was a high school senior, Kim had returned to work. But her nervousness got in the way. She had to quit her job as an administrative assistant at a university, because of her nerves. This upset Kim. She had always taken pride in her work. Before the kids were born, she had been an administrative assistant to the CEO of a large company. But on returning to work, after twenty years as a mom, Kim found the world had changed.

"They wanted me to learn how to use the computer, a program they called Excel. I really wanted to. I tried but I couldn't. The phone would ring. My boss would want something. My kids would call me with questions. Interruptions all the time. And the pressure. Everyone wants things right away. Before the kids were born, I used to work for just one person. In this new job, there are six people I'm supposed to take care of. I don't

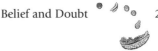

know how I can do it. The computer is supposed to help, but it doesn't. It just makes me nervous and slows me down.

"I tried one of those on-line seminars. But I couldn't follow it. The way they explained things confused me."

Gradually, inexorably, Kim lost confidence in herself. She started to worry about work. She had trouble sleeping. When she woke up in the morning, she had a knot in her stomach as she thought about going to work. She began having headaches.

Then her son, always a lively child, began to have trouble. He had found a girlfriend. He began to come home late and to miss school. Then, one night, he was arrested for having beer in his car.

"That did it for me," Kim said. "I became obsessed with books about teenage boys. I read everything. Watched every show I could. And it left me feeling like a bad mom. Like I had failed him somehow. That was when the anxiety attacks started at work. I would be sitting at my computer, trying to learn that foolish program, my boss would call, and then the attacks hit. I would shake, my heart raced and I had to get some air. It happened one too many times, so I quit."

Kim was out of balance. Her belief in herself was shaken. Flooded by demands from a world that had changed, she doubted herself and her abilities. The result, riddled by worry, unable to sleep, feeling sick every day, was that she withdrew. When Kim consulted me, she was spending her day at home, doing housework and avoiding social contact.

"Every time the phone rings, I jump," she told me.

The first goal of Kim's treatment was to help her to feel less nervous. For a time, she took a medication that blocked her nervousness. At least she slept better and felt calmer, but it was

*only a start. We supplemented this with some exercise and with
some training in relaxation techniques.*

*"I'm pretty sure that I can stay physically calm," she told me,
"but I'm still too nervous to work. I'm afraid I'll fail again."*

*We talked for a time about her interests, what she liked and
what she was good at. As the oldest of six children, born to a
Christian family in Kentucky, caring for children and members
of her family had been her life. Her family believed in the
Christian ideal of taking care of others before you take care of
yourself.*

*"It's what I do. I know kids and people. I can do that," Kim
said. It became clear that she felt best when helping other
people out, especially kids. That is what had drawn her to being
an administrative assistant. But as the job became more technologically oriented, Kim doubted her ability. Her thoughts
became filled with fear and worry. She dreaded work, having
convinced herself that she would fail. She began to accuse herself of being too slow, too stupid and too shy for work. She
doubted herself.*

*The next step for Kim was to restore her belief in herself. I
referred her to a cognitive therapist, who helped Kim learn how
to talk positively to herself. Gradually, Kim learned how to
replace the negative, worried dialogue in her mind with meaningful words of encouragement. She learned how to actively
draw on her natural people skills, to trust that she would know
the right thing to do. Taking notice of the warm and pleasant
reactions that she produced in people who she was helping,
Kim regained confidence in her abilities. It was a good fit with
her religious beliefs, too. Each Sunday, as she sat in church,
singing hymns, enjoying the ritual of the service, Kim reflected*

on the importance to her of caring for others, as a good Christian should.

What really made this work for Kim was how much she liked and trusted her therapist. She believed in him. And each time she found herself in a situation that made her nervous, Kim actively recalled the steps he had taught her.

Kim's Rules for Managing Doubt

1. *Movement helps. She should calm herself physically, breathe, relax and move around.*
2. *Allow her people skills to pull her through.*
3. *Follow Christian principles in helping others.*
4. *Talk positively to herself as Dr. Black (her therapist) had taught.*
5. *Gain strength from attending church services.*

Feeling better, calm and free of anxiety, Kim was able to find a job as a teacher's aide in her local school.

"I just love the kids," she told me.

And, turning her attention to her teenage son, she taught him what she had learned about talking positively to himself. She taught him how to be more self-assured with girls. More confident with himself, he didn't need beer to get the courage to go on a date.

Kim reestablished balance in her life by strengthening her belief, in herself, in her body and in her faith.

A Society of Doubt

When anything seems possible, when you can do anything at any time, it can be difficult to know what to do. It is a strange time, when scientific certainty is everywhere, examining every detail of life, attempting to explain the unexplainable and in the process, introducing doubt into the fabric of existence. It is a time of breathtaking discoveries and it is a time of penetrating questions. Here are some "beliefs" that had been obvious truths to our ancestors, that science has proven wrong in the last two hundred years:

- Man can't fly.
- The world is flat.
- Exposure to bad air causes infection.
- The world is made of air, water and fire.
- Riding a horse is the fastest way to travel.
- Time and distance are universal constants.
- It's not possible to communicate quickly with someone in a distant place.

Science and technology progress through doubt. Science is advanced by disproving theories, by raising questions, by doubting. Then, through a process of breaking a problem down into small parts, gathering facts and by conducting analysis, the factual truth becomes apparent. Science gives us answers by systematically raising doubts.

We are all better off for all of this inquiry. Now we have

airplanes, telephones and antibiotics. We have heat and lights. We have fantastic machines that can perform unimaginable tasks, like putting thousands of circuits on the head of a pin. We celebrate the success of science. We live with the success of science and technology. We are healthier because of the success of science. And, because doubt propels science forward, we have learned to doubt. Because the very things that seem certain and apparent today may well be disproven tomorrow.

We have become a culture of doubt, a society of doubt and disbelief. No longer do we have the bedrock faith of our ancestors. We doubt the human fundamentals that existed, with no questions asked, until two hundred years ago. We doubt basic human facts, those rhythms that guided life over millions of years, natural human rhythms that produce balance have come under question.

How much has it changed for us? Consider this. The Egyptian culture existed for five thousand years as a culture of belief. The rhythm of life was driven by the changing of the seasons. Each year, the predictable flood of the Nile River set the pattern of life: when the Egyptians planted crops, when they harvested, when they held feasts and religious festivals, all were ordered by the annual cycle of the Nile River floods. And in this cycle grew a society of belief. There was a ruling class to guide the country, a class of priests to administer the rituals of belief, a soldier class to defend the country, a class of merchants to distribute the harvest and a class of farmers to grow the food.

Was it a perfect society? No, not by any measure. But it

was predictable. It was a human society driven by the natural rules of belief, by belief in the reproductive cycles of nature, in the hierarchy of work, in the safety and security of the culture and in the belief that a higher power was guiding life in Egypt. If you could live with an Egyptian family of 4000 B.C. and compare it to an Egyptian family three thousand years later, you would find that the pattern of life, the circumstances of life, were unchanged over the intervening 3000 years.

Compare this to our society. My mother-in-law was raised on a farm in Wisconsin about seventy years ago, one generation ago. On her family's farm, there was no phone, no electricity, no running water, no automobiles. Heat was provided by a wood stove. To go to school, my mother-in-law had to live with cousins in Sturgeon Bay, away from her family for weeks at a time, because the school in Sturgeon Bay was twenty miles from the farm.

Contrast this to my family. One simple fact tells the tale. Each day, I drive twenty miles to work, and I bring my daughter, Nora, who is five years old, with me, to attend a preschool that is twenty miles from home. And each day, Nora is back home by 12:30! This set of circumstances would have been unimaginable to my mother-in-law during her childhood.

In our society, there has been more dramatic change in just seventy years than there was in the entire five thousand years of Egyptian culture. In just seventy years, the circumstances of life have changed so much, that the only constant is change and doubt.

It is no wonder we doubt. It is now the natural order of

things. With the wonders of science, there is no reason to accept external limits. Through the inexorable progress of scientific inquiry, new opportunities, new technologies, new solutions to old problems are developed every day.

The scientific revolution of the last two hundred years has given us many wonderful technologies. It is the best of times to be alive. But the principles of the scientific revolution lead right to doubt. Flooded daily with the excitement, the possibilities and the certainties of modern life, we have begun to raise questions about some very basic human needs. You have seen the balance problems that result in the earlier chapters of this book.

Because we can work and play twenty-four hours per day, we doubt the need for sleep. Because we can drive or fly to go where we want to go, we doubt the need for movement and exercise. Because of the abundance of modern life, we doubt the need to plan for and to regulate our appetites. Because we see images of people all day long, and because we can communicate electronically, we doubt the need to be with people. Because we are flooded with ideas, images and information, we doubt ourselves.

Balance problems in modern life come from doubting your own natural rules and from doubting your own natural rhythms and flow. Balance problems come from believing the stimulating, dramatic urgency of modern life, instead of believing in yourself and your natural rhythms as a human being.

Modern life deals a double blow to belief. The urgency, the "illusion of certainty" that gets right to your brain's alarm systems causes you to live in a state of nervousness and worry. But the culture of doubt in which we live then casts doubt on the very things that each of us needs to quiet our fears, to soothe our worries, to help us to feel safe, secure and confident. When you do not believe, accept and act on your needs as a member of the human race, when you do not live within the natural rules of your body, your brain and your mind, the price you pay is balance.

The good news is that you can live with a healthy balance by practicing the natural rules of belief.

Your program of balance all comes together with belief.

Belief Balances Doubt

There is mystery to life. Miracles and magic, too. Despite our technological advances, there is still so much that we do not understand. So much that we cannot reduce to particles, to forces, to mathematical equations. And when you face the unknowable with a firm belief, instead of fear and worry, you live with mystery, miracles and magic. Belief balances doubt, by guiding you away from the dark corners of your mind, away from the black recesses of fear, turning you instead to the hopeful magic, the creative mysteries and the inspiring miracles of life.

With our ancient brains, developed in a simpler time, it is likely to always be this way. There are some events that we cannot understand. Like love between two people. Like the miracle of birth. Like the mystery of the way we change and grow throughout life. Like the miracle of creativity that brings us a new idea. Like the simple miracle of waking up each morning to greet the possibilities of a new day.

For the factors are so complex and varied, the calculus of life so elegant, that we cannot reduce all of the events of life to a logical assembly of facts, with clear rules and procedures. And so, we must believe.

The human brain was created in such a way that belief makes life possible, in the face of the mystery, the magic and the miracles of everyday life. In the workings of your brain, a strong system of belief provides a reassuring organization to the flow of your thought, your emotion and your mental energy. Belief helps us understand.

That is why humans drew reverential pictures of animals in southern France, 50,000 years ago.

That is why each society of people has constructed temples of worship, from the decaying ruins of Machu Picchu to the dazzling temples of the Mormons in Salt Lake City and Washington.

That is why in the British Islands, prehistoric man moved impossibly huge slabs of rock to construct Stonehenge, a temple of the solstice.

That is why today, despite the scientific certainties of our technology, there is an upsurge of belief, in organized religion; in mystic forms of New Age belief; in the magic cycles of reincarnation and in the hopeful mysteries of spirit life, mediums and communication with the dead. A Gallup poll in 1996 found 70 percent of Americans believe in angels.

Of course we believe, we have to. In the face of the unknowable, it is belief that guides. In fact, your brain is constructed to believe. It is part of being human.

One hundred thousand years ago, as language developed in the human race, as complex social groups emerged, as we humans learned to think, to create and to care for one another, we started to believe. You see, belief is an organizing principle of the mind. Belief is what scientists call a "meta" program, i.e., a program that organizes and conducts other programs. In the brain, your system of beliefs guides you; it activates and coordinates all other parts of the brain; telling you when to be social and when to fight, when to be happy and when to be sad, when to help out and when to condemn, when to take action and when to wait. Your system of belief tells you what is right and what is wrong. Belief organizes and coordinates all of the systems of your mind, into a rhythmic, harmonious and balanced life.

At the level of your neurological systems, belief exists through the cooperation of all parts of your neocortex. Your brain files away knowledge of organizing beliefs that are composed of elements produced by all parts of the brain. In the workings of your brain, a belief is assembled from memory, from visual images, from important words and phrases, from guiding mental processes (operational rules), from patterns of emotion, and from models of behavior learned from important people. These elements are assembled into a set of principles that guide you.

To give you a feel for how this operates, consider this scenario. Imagine that I am trying to help a woman, who has a condition that is presenting in a way that is confusing and new to me. Imagine, if you will, that you could listen to my brain provide me with guidance, based on my belief in the principles of medical practice. You would hear something like this:

"This patient is in distress. Her symptoms seem confusing. But what matters most is to reassure her that you can provide her with help. Conduct an examination as you have learned to do, then tell her what you think; that is always helpful. Provide her with something to help her to feel better. Later when you have time, you can research her condition to come up with more answers. If there is still confusion about the cause of her distress, then you can always send her for consultation. But remember to always reassure her that you will try your best to help, because that is what matters most."

Now let's create an everyday example to see how belief works. In this example, you are trying to cook dinner when you realize that your ten-year-old son is playing video games instead of doing his homework. You are pressed for time, and you have already spoken to your son once. Your instincts are to yell at your son and to shut off the computer, or to just ignore the whole thing. But drawing on your beliefs about being a parent, a different scenario emerges. If you could listen to the language of your brain, here is what you might hear:

"Billy is doing it again! I don't have time to deal with him. But he seems to be having trouble settling down. I wonder if there is a problem at school, or maybe something is bothering him. That has happened before. Last time he had trouble it was because the teacher had been critical of him in class. I better talk with him, to see if I can help. It breaks my heart to think he could be upset. I'll turn the stove on low, and spend a few minutes talking to him. Dinner can wait; he is more important. Besides, if I can help him to sort this out, we'll all feel better."

In both examples, a set of beliefs provided guidance in the face of uncertainty. You can see that the belief is made up of the coordinated actions of different brain functions: memory, language, feeling, energy and movement, organized into some guiding principles. The result is an action or behavior that feels right, and that successfully deals with the situation.

A strong system of belief guides you when you confront the inevitable mysteries and magic of life, whether that mystery comes from your own confusion about what you feel or who you are, or from the outside world, when circumstances are ambiguous and unnerving.

Belief, as I am defining it here, is not just about religion, although religion is certainly an important form of belief. In the workings of the brain, belief is a set of principles that guide you. You could speak of values, morals and ethics in the same way that I am referring to belief. You could also speak of religion, law and civics in the same way. Or you could speak of practices, discipline or professionalism. All of these words refer to belief: a set of principles, learned from a power larger than yourself, transmitted from person to person, that guides your behavior and your life.

Consider these questions as a way of further defining belief.

Why would I let myself be awakened repeatedly, in the middle of the night, to talk with strangers on behalf of a patient? Because I believe in the ethics and practice of medicine.

Why would you dive in the street to save your child from an onrushing truck, defying the logic of your own self-preservation? Because you believe in the sanctity of life and in your God-given role as a parent.

Why would you restrict what you eat and exercise to lose weight? Because you believe your doctor when she tells you that losing weight and exercising is healthy for you.

Why would you leave the comfort of your home in a driving November rain to vote for someone you have never met? Because you believe in being a good citizen.

Why would you get down on your knees and pray for strength and guidance? Because you believe in God.

Belief guides you. When it is just not possible to know the facts, or to be certain about a plan of action; when you can see conflicting positions or irreconcilable differences and you still must make a decision; when, in the flow of your day, you have choices to make; when life presents you with a new opportunity in uncharted waters; in the face of the mysteries, magic and miracles of life, belief guides you.

You can tell that belief is powerful by the effects of strong belief on your health. Those with strong beliefs have been found by medical researchers to get these benefits:

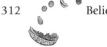

- less hypertension
- lower incidence of heart disease
- improved relationships with people
- a better chance of having a healthy baby
- less depression and anxiety
- better survival from cancer.

Those with strong beliefs have better, longer marriages. Those with strong beliefs are happier and more optimistic. Those with strong beliefs have more financial success.

Like an all-purpose tonic for your body and soul, belief activates and coordinates beneficial mental and physical processes that leave you in a healthy balance.

The Practice of Belief

Although belief helps you tap into the wisdom of powers larger than yourself, the practice of belief is still a fundamentally human activity. And like any human activity, the practice of belief can be learned; the practice of belief can be strengthened. You can live with passion, with the excitement and possibility of our technologic age while staying in balance, if you follow the practice of belief.

Using the practice of belief helps you counter the worry, nervousness and unease that comes from living in our modern society of doubt. The framework is familiar to you by now from previous chapters. Using natural rules of balance, rules that are based on the way that your brain and mind is made, you engage the higher centers of your brain, to balance the energy and stimulation from the lower centers. In this case, our society of doubt leads you to live in a constant state of stressful alarm, poor sleep, nervous tension, worry and anxiety. All of this because your ancient brain is reacting as it must to the constant stream of new information and demand. You balance this with the natural rules of belief; these rules allow the higher centers of your brain to function naturally, in the way they were created, following a healthy practice of belief. In doing so, you calm and quiet the alarm systems from your ancient brain. You live in balance.

Through the study of man, anthropologists have learned about the sustaining practices of belief. Through fossil records, historical artifacts and by sophisticated genetic studies, biologists have learned about the human development of belief. Through studying the complex ways that brain and mind interact, cognitive neuroscientists have been able to describe the pathways of belief.

From all of this learning and study, it is possible to decipher the practices of belief; those natural human rules that produce a balance of belief and doubt. The essence of the natural rules for the balance of belief and doubt is producing a state of mind where all other mental processes are smoothly coordinated into a pleasing pattern of action and behavior. You can learn these practices. You may already know them. And when you apply the rules, when you follow the practices of belief, then you will be able to confidently make sense of your life.

Let's review the rules that researchers have found to produce a strong and calming practice of belief in man.

The Natural Rules of Belief

Rule #1: Talk to Yourself in a Helpful Manner

Whether you call it prayer, or affirmation, or positive thinking, or even cognitive reframing, the process of talking to yourself in a helpful manner is the fundamental practice of belief. Many helpful religious practices are based on the idea of using the words of God to help yourself to learn to talk positively to yourself. The powerful psychotherapy, called cognitive therapy, is based on learning how to talk to yourself in a helpful manner. St. Paul, one of the founding fathers of Christianity, taught the early Christians that the foundation of firm belief is learning to talk to yourself. You can hear it in this quote.

> Finally brethren, whatsoever things are true, whatsoever things are honest, whatsoever things are just, whatsoever things are pure, whatsoever things are lovely, whatsoever things are of good report; if there be any virtue, if there be any praise, *think on these things.*
>
> St. Paul to the Philippians, 4:8

One of the best modern examples is the way that Alcoholics Anonymous uses positive self-talk to strengthen belief in the Twelve-Step program. This organization, the most successful approach to treating alcoholism, is a program based in the practice of belief. One of the basic tools in AA is learning to talk to yourself in a helpful manner.

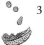

AA literature and AA meetings are filled with sayings, aphorisms and ideas that the members adopt and use to ward off the temptation to drink. The sayings make belief in the power of AA even stronger. Famous examples (examples that are so famous that they have become part of our general patterns of speech) include: "one day at a time," "keep it simple," "submit to your higher power."

And it is based in good science, too. When you talk to yourself, the words and phrases activate other brain functions linked to the words you choose. A helpful phrase might link a memory, an action and an emotion into a unified whole. At the level of the nerve cell, the wiring of these functions is actually connected to the brain systems producing the words. When you talk in a helpful manner to yourself, you organize these brain systems into a unified flow.

Talking to yourself in a helpful manner can include praise, encouragement, guidance, affirmation or explanation. By talking to yourself in a helpful manner, you confirm your beliefs and you help yourself to act in accordance with those beliefs. By talking to yourself in a helpful manner, you balance doubt.

Rule #2: Guide Yourself with Helpful Images

Pictures, images, statues, buildings, even ceremonial clothing, all are visual symbols that guide and strengthen belief. Just as your brain uses words and language to guide belief, so, too, can your brain use images. It is a right-brain type of language. Equally powerful, using a similar mental mechanism as language, guiding yourself with helpful visual representations is one of the practices of belief.

Think about it for a minute, and you will see what I mean. Churches are filled with pictures, statues and furnishings that are the visual symbols of belief. I will never forget the colorful robes, the golden crosses, the vivid stations of the cross, the stained glass windows that symbolized belief in the Catholic churches of my youth.

It is not limited to religion. Have you ever been to a sports hall of fame? There you will find room after room of pictures and statues that represent our beliefs about the purity and power of sport.

At universities, you will find the same. Statues and pictures that represent belief in higher learning and the power of education.

The visual images need not be static. The memory of a person or group of people in the process of performing a meaningful act can be a powerful tool for strengthening belief. I can still recall favorite professors in medical school, in the act of examining a patient. I draw on those images to guide me now; the images help me follow my beliefs about the practice of medicine.

This practice makes good brain sense. Your right brain learns visually, by creating a mental image of someone or something. By doing so, your brain is taking in the whole picture and not just a small component. Abstract, conceptual learning is felt to be a right-brain function that uses pictures and images as its particular form of thought. When you guide yourself with helpful images, you are helping your right brain to process the abstract notion of belief, the whole picture of belief, not just the words. Visual images are a powerful learning tool that help you to carry out a complex action according to a guiding set of principles. This is especially helpful when the principles may be too complex to follow in recipe fashion, step by step. Most belief systems are complex, hence using visual images will help you strengthen your practice of belief when words alone are not enough.

To use images in the practice of belief, you need only to recall a mental image that symbolizes an important aspect of your belief system. The image will serve the purpose of activating and coordinating your brain's function, into a pattern of thought, feeling and behavior that is guided by belief.

Rule # 3: Accept Guiding Principles from Outside of Yourself

Whether it is following the moral teachings or your religion or the Twelve Steps of Alcoholics Anonymous, or the ethics of your profession, accepting guiding principles from outside of yourself is an important practice of belief. When you do, you can take comfort in the notion that your actions are following principles set out by a power greater than yourself.

The human brain was created to learn complex patterns of social behavior, from parents, from peers, from our elders and from the accumulated wisdom of others. This function allowed our ancestors to operate in social groupings, surviving better as a group than as lonely individuals.

What started out as a biologic survival mechanism turned into a defining human characteristic. The ability to understand abstract principles of behavior, guiding group activity, turned into the foundation of belief. The human mind readily grasps ethical, moral and religious principles, understanding the meaning, translating the abstract principles into rules for living.

Guiding principles from outside of yourself provide you with a clear road map for your life; they resolve ambiguity, provide reassurance, help you move confidently in the face of the unknown.

It makes good sense. Whether it is spiritual guidance, or the practical guidance that comes from a code of ethics, the message is the same: "Set aside your doubts and worries. Have faith. Here are some time-tested principles that have worked for others; use them to guide you and you will benefit as those before you have."

Accepting guidance from outside yourself helps you in two clear ways. It is a form of belief that directly counters worry. If you are worried about something in life, actively recalling what you have learned from a force that is larger than yourself—your religious practice, your moral code, your ethics—your guiding principles will stop the worry, replacing it with a clear understanding of how to act. And it sets up a healthy process in your mind; following trusted principles in which you have great faith is calming and reassuring. The higher centers in your brain, under the influence of your guiding principles, send calming messages to the lower center of your brain, telling the alarm centers in your brain stem, "Don't worry, we know what to do, everything is under control, it will all work out for the best." It builds confidence in yourself. It builds confidence in your life.

Rule #4: Belong to a Group of Like-Minded People

In this book, you have seen the ways that close relationships with people are essential to a healthy balance. In part, this is because of the important effect that close relationships have on belief. When you belong to a group of like-minded people, you become part of a society of belief. Fed by the human contact, your beliefs are nourished and strengthened. Each time you gather together, you strengthen the bond of belief, through mutual support and encouragement, through hearing the stories of belief from your fellow members, through the energy of a shared emotional experience, through a process of mutual education and guidance with each person contributing thoughts on how they understand the principles of belief; your beliefs are strengthened.

It has worked well over the millions of years of human existence. Groups of people, banding together in common purpose, living in harmony, accomplishing great things.

Our country was created as a society of belief: one nation, under God, with each person possessing inalienable rights to freedom and the pursuit of happiness. This is an elegant statement of belief. Together as a society of belief, we have prospered.

The lesson to each of us is to find a group of like-minded people, create a society of belief, to balance doubt, to strengthen your principles of belief, to live in balance.

Rule #5: Follow the Steps Set Out by a Trusted Leader

Throughout the history of man, there have been individuals, women and men, who are accorded a special status in human society. Wise men, shamans, priests, doctors, seers, gurus and patriarchs all serve the same purpose: to lead by example, to embody the principles of belief and, through deep wisdom, to guide the actions of human society.

A trusted leader is a powerful influence on the practice of belief. Why? It is because of the way we are made. From the moment you are born, your brain is deeply imprinted by lessons that are learned through the actions of someone you care about. The stronger the feeling and the greater the trust in that person, the more powerfully the lesson is learned. And if the person leading has wisdom, a deep and special knowledge, the product of unique gifts, burnished through years of hard work and deprivation, then that leader becomes a powerful emotional presence, the living symbol of a system of belief.

Listen to this quote from *Persuasion and Healing*. It beautifully summarizes the role of a trusted leader in a community of believers.

> The intercession of people united in love for Christ . . . and the laying on of hands . . . by a priest or minister or other person who is the contact point . . . of a beloved, believing and united community standing behind him and supporting his ministration to a patient who has been taught to understand the true nature of Christian faith . . . is the true ministry of the Church.

When you follow the steps set out by a trusted leader, you strengthen belief through the power of your personal relationship with the leader. This process can heal. It can guide, it can explain. It can instruct. In a way, it is exactly in tune with the benefits of accepting guidance from a power greater than yourself except, in this instance, it is a person who shows the way. The personal, emotional connection to the leader makes the practice of belief even stronger.

Following a spiritual leader has been a human practice for as long as humans have walked on this planet. But the practice is not limited to just spiritual pursuits. The power of this special relationship can strengthen your beliefs about any activity that matters to you. A teacher can be a trusted leader. A therapist, too. A mentor is a type of trusted leader. And so is a coach. What makes this work are three things:

- The leader is a model for the principles of belief.
- The leader has acquired special knowledge.
- You trust and believe in the leader as a person.

Find someone you trust, follow the steps they recommend and your practice of belief will be strengthened. It is a natural rule for balancing doubt.

Rule #6: Perform Helpful Rituals

To live according to your principles of belief, you must, of course, take action in a manner that is in harmony with your belief. Your actions and your behavior become the living expression of your belief. Your actions express your

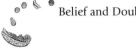

belief, and since your mind works as a two-way street, your actions reinforce and strengthen your belief.

Helpful rituals are central to belief. The actions of the ritual express the central tenets of belief. As you take part in the ritual, the relationship with your fellow believers and with the leader, the sights and sounds of the ritual and the movement of the ritual all activate neural structures that underlie belief. Ritual is the *action* of belief. Ritual is one way that you and your brain learn about belief; as you take part in the ritual you are really practicing and refining all of the mental pathways necessary to support belief; these are pathways for social belonging, for emotional connections, for positive beliefs about yourself and your future. Rituals commonly involve movement, singing or chanting and the telling of an important story because that is how your brain processes thought. The ritual serves to confirm and validate the underlying structure and practice of belief.

Examples abound.

The communion ritual in the Christian faith celebrates Christ's sacrifice on behalf of mankind. The communion ritual expresses belief in the divinity of Christ, and it validates the Christian ethic of putting the interests of your fellow man before your own.

The ritual of bar mitzvah in the Jewish faith celebrates the coming of age of male children. The ritual is also an expression of and a validation of the belief that each adult is part of a community of law and that it is the responsibility of each adult to live within the laws of the Jewish community of faith.

To cite a more mundane example, the annual physical exam is a ritual of modern life. It is an expression of the belief that modern medicine can prevent disease, and that the physicians possess the knowledge to guide healthy behavior. Having an annual physical, in part, confirms the healing power of medicine and the physician.

The practice of psychotherapy is effective in healing emotional problems, in part because of the ritual involved. The ritual of psychotherapy, the weekly visit to the therapist's office, the ritual discussion of emotional events, the dispensing of insight and advice by the therapist all are expressions of the belief that there are psychological insights that can heal by reordering emotional life. The rituals of psychotherapy confirm and validate that belief.

You can strengthen your practice of belief by using elements of helpful ritual.

One man I know, a professional baseball player, strengthened his belief in his skill by performing a series of rituals: touching the bat to the ground in a certain way, throwing the ball in a particular way and the same number of times, adjusting his clothing in just the same way before stepping up to the plate.

A successful investor that I know strengthens his belief in his ability to make correct investment decisions by checking a model investment portfolio four times per day, at the same time each day 8:00 A.M., 10:00 A.M., 2:00 P.M. and 4:00 P.M. It is, of course a good practice for an investor. But this ritual also is the expression of the belief that he is careful investor who can judge the market when given enough timely information.

Use helpful ritual to confirm and validate your positive view of the world. Use helpful ritual to strengthen your practice of belief and to help you effectively balance doubt.

Rule #7: Use Special Places

The Chinese call it "feng shui," Neurologists call it "environmental dependence." Psychologists refer to it as being "stimulus bound." It does not matter what your perspective or how you label it, there is direct and potent connection between special places and the smooth functioning of belief, created in harmony with the biology of your brain and mind.

Religious believers, through the ages, have demonstrated the belief-enhancing power of special places through the construction of temples, churches and shrines. In the secular world, a trip to Washington, D.C., to view the uniquely powerful national monuments, will convince you of the way that special places enhance belief. Our national monuments in Washington, through their beauty and emotional power, strengthen the central beliefs of this country. Courts of law, both local and national, always built to look solid and imposing, are really temples of belief, dedicated to strengthening belief in the rule of law. Universities, especially the libraries of universities, are built to have the feel of wisdom, the security of knowledge. These buildings are special places where belief in learning is strengthened while being carried out.

When researchers study belief, they find that place or environmental setting is a powerful determinant of belief. The same neurochemical reaction can be interpreted by test subjects as excitement, happiness, anger or fear depending on the elements of place. In the mind's language of survival, having a sense of place helps you line up the proper feelings, thoughts and behaviors, in harmony with the needs of your environment, so you are better prepared to survive. You may recall this as a fundamental principle of balance from chapter 2; your brain must live in harmony with the external circumstances of life. It is an active principle of balance for living organisms from single-cell bacteria, right up to we complex humans.

Of course your environment matters. And when you are in a special place, it can strengthen and influence those guiding principles of life called belief.

You can use special places to reinforce your belief. It may be a special place by the ocean that reinforces your belief that things will turn out all right; it may be a corner of your home, a place where you believe you can get work done; it may be your church where you are filled with belief in the goodness of mankind; it may be a restaurant where you and your husband went while dating, where you believe in the strength of your relationship.

What matters here is that the place has the feel of your belief. When you are in your special place, the sights, the sounds, the feel and the rhythms of the place activate the complex patterns of belief in your mind and in your heart. Use special places to strengthen your belief, to balance doubt.

It is natural and healthy to believe. And there are steps you can take to strengthen your beliefs. That is how you achieve balance in a society of doubt, by following a practice of belief. You apply these "meta" rules to your entire life, to guide you in all aspects of your life, to make sense of what you do, to help you to live in rhythmic harmony with the circumstances of your life.

Listen to Nancy's story about regaining balance through the practice of belief.

"Nothing I Do Seems Good Enough"

Her kids were twelve and fourteen when Nancy first consulted me.

"I worry all the time that I'm a terrible mother," Nancy revealed. "No matter what I do, it never seems like enough. Tracey is just starting to discover boys. She's on the computer all the time. That instant message thing on AOL. So she doesn't listen to me. And Billy needs help with his schoolwork. He gets so frustrated and angry. I've tried everything, and he still yells at me. The only way I get peace is if I let him play video games. My husband is no help. He just asks me what I do all day, as if I sat at home just watching soap operas.

"I can't stand it. I feel so upset with myself. That was how the drinking started. After the kids went to bed, out came the bottle of wine to help me to relax."

Nancy's drinking had gotten out of hand. Two glasses of wine had become a bottle. One bottle had become two. When

Nancy began to have a glass of wine before lunch to "make the day go better," she knew that she was in trouble. It all came to a head when her husband came home early one day to find Nancy asleep on the couch, an empty wine bottle on the coffee table, the television blaring away in the background. Brian insisted that she get help.

We talked about how it happened.

"I quit my job when my mother got sick. It wasn't a big job, just helping out as office manager at a real estate office. About twenty hours per week while the kids were at school. I liked it though. I loved the contact with the customers, so excited about buying a home, you know. It was fun to keep the office running. But Mom had a stroke; she couldn't walk anymore. She needed me. So I quit to help her. I didn't know that it would take over my life the way it did."

Always somewhat irascible, after the stroke Nancy's mom became angry, demanding and extremely critical of Nancy. To be helpful to her mom, Nancy had started to carry a cell phone. The calls were always the same. Minutes after Nancy left her side, her mom would call to make a demand or to complain; something that Nancy had done for her wasn't right. Buying the wrong brand of soap, being late with her medicine, not answering her call fast enough.

"It really got to me," Nancy said. "Here I was just about killing myself to help her, and all she could do was complain. It's the story of my life. In her eyes, I've never been good enough. Not like my sister, who walks on water."

The rest of her life did not stop because she had chosen to take care of her ill mother. In between trips to her mom's house, there were appointments for the kids, shopping for her home, *cleaning the house, helping with homework. All the while, Nancy tried to be the best mom that she could.*

But it did get under her skin. She began to feel like she was failing. Every request, to her, felt like an indication that she had done something wrong. She became nervous and tense. She couldn't sleep. Then she started to drink.

"The worry stops when I drink," Nancy told me. "There is that warm feeling that comes with the first glass of wine, it kind of feels as though things will be all right in a minute or two. And if I drink enough, then I can sleep."

Nancy had to stop drinking. She had started to avoid her kids. She and Brian never talked anymore. She no longer taught Sunday school, or helped raise money for the church. Little by little, her life was collapsing inward. What was left were her mother's demands, her worries and the alcohol.

Our first step on Nancy's path to balance was to have her become involved with Alcoholics Anonymous. With her husband's firm insistence, Nancy quit drinking, replacing her nightly glasses of wine with a trip to an AA meeting. There she met a friend who became her sponsor. The spiritual power of AA began to take hold.

"I've met a great friend at the meetings. Alice has been in the program for ten years. The things that she knows . . . she tells me what to expect, how to follow the program and how it's worked for her. I like her a lot."

As Nancy worked her AA program, a change came over her.

"It's a funny thing, but I feel more confident," she said. "You'd kind of expect the opposite, what with all the drunk-a-logues and the stories about alcoholism. But the things that Alice tells me really stick. I'm finding that I think of those things when I'm

with my mom. Like, one day at a time, and giving myself over to a higher power. And you know, I'm starting to question the relationship I had with my mom when I was a girl."

The middle of five children, all born in a six-year time span, Nancy recalled a childhood filled with noise, chaos and confusion. Her mother, already a demanding and critical person, became more so under the pressure of raising five kids. With her naturally sweet disposition, eager to help her stressed-out mom, Nancy assumed more and more of the household chores for her mother. She would cheerfully cook and clean, and as she grew older, Nancy took on a mother role for her siblings. But instead of thanks, her mom only became more critical.

"I came to believe that I was good for nothing and that I only got by thanks to the grace of God."

Her only peace came at church. The familiar ritual of the service, the rhythmic beauty of the choir music, the reassuring words of the sermon, the pleasant warmth of sitting in a church pew with people who believed, as she did.

I encouraged Nancy to get involved again with church. She started to attend Sunday services and instead of volunteering to raise money, she joined the church choir.

"I love the gentle beauty of the music," she said. "I feel good when I'm singing. And you know, it feels right to be part of the choir. We sing well, and I fit. It reminds me of the happy times."

Still, there was more work to do. Although she was no longer drinking, Nancy was still convinced that she was not a good mother, that somehow she would fail her kids.

We talked of her dad. A good man, he was a clerk in the courts. To make ends meet for his big family, in the evenings and on weekends he worked as a mason, fixing walls, painting chimneys and building walks. He could not be home enough. One day, rummaging through an old photo album, Nancy found a picture. It was she and her dad, at a birthday party for her brother. Her dad was leaning over, whispering in her ear.

When she found that picture, a wave of emotion swept over her. She remembered her dad saying, "I'm sorry to have to ask you to do these things, but I need you."

Unsure of what to make of this, Nancy began to visit her father's grave in the family plot. He had died when she was eighteen. Bringing flowers twice a week, Nancy found comfort in her brief visits. As she stood by his grave, placing the flowers by the granite headstone, her thoughts turned to her dad. She began to recall the warm praise that he had for her, whenever they had a few moments alone. Nancy recalled his words, "I ask you to take care of things because you are so good at it. Your mother needs your help." Each time she visited his grave, Nancy felt her dad's presence, and she began to feel better. She carried the picture of her dad with her wherever she went. Over time, she learned to remember her dad's words to her. Her doubts about herself began to fade.

Nancy started to take her mom to Sunday service with her. Resistant at first, her mom eventually took pleasure in the hopeful joy of the celebration. After church, they sat and talked. And it helped. Nancy confirmed her belief in herself as her mom opened up, sharing stories about Nancy's childhood.

More relaxed about herself, Nancy found it easier to care for her kids. She could accept their different ways, trusting that if she loved them enough, they would be okay.

Nancy found a peaceful balance through the practice of belief. Here is a list of the ways that she applied the rules for balancing doubt with healthy belief.

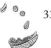

Nancy's Rules for the Practice of Belief

1. *Talk positively to herself. Remember her dad's words, remember the simple affirmations of AA, talk to herself as she learned from Alice.*
2. *Guide herself with positive images. Carry a picture of her dad. Remember an image of the celebration of Mass.*
3. *Accept guiding principles from outside herself. Live her life as a good Christian. Follow the Twelve Steps of Alcoholics Anonymous.*
4. *Belong to a group of like-minded people. Go to church. Join the church choir. Join Alcoholics Anonymous.*
5. *Follow a trusted leader. Listen to the words of advice from Alice. Follow the teachings of Christ through the words of her minister.*
6. *Perform helpful rituals by attending AA meetings, attending church services, singing in the choir and visiting her father's grave.*
7. *Use special places including church and her dad's gravesite.*

By following a practice of belief, Nancy was able to balance the doubt she had lived with; the doubt that came from the circumstances of her life. When she strengthened her belief, Nancy was able to live as she needed to and wanted to, while at the same time maintaining a peaceful balance.

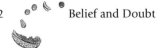

Personal Balance
Comes Together with Belief

Are you wondering how you can make this all work? Are you unsure how to establish a healthy balance when modern life is filled with stimulation, excitement and passion? Are you confused about how to follow the rules of balance outlined in these chapters?

The answer is belief. The pathway to a natural and healthy balance flows through the practice of belief. The seven rules for the practice of belief are the rules that guide the operation of your mind. The rules guiding the practice of belief are the operating principles of the mind.

Here are the natural rules of balance for strengthening belief, to establish and maintain a healthy practice of belief.

Belief and Doubt Self-Test

Take this test to see if you are out of balance. If you answered yes to two or more questions, you may have a problem with the balance of belief and doubt. To improve your balance, you should try to incorporate the rules in this chapter as well as the tips to follow.

1.	Do you often find yourself worrying even when you know things will turn out all right?	yes	no
2.	Do you often feel flooded by so much information that you don't know who or what to believe?	yes	no
3.	Do you feel that you lack confidence or faith in yourself?	yes	no
4.	Do you feel that money, power or fame matters more to most people than ethics, values or morals?	yes	no

Score_____

Tips to Balance Belief and Doubt

Here is a list of tips to help you with the practice of belief. Use these tips and enjoy the benefit of strong, sustaining beliefs; belief that guides, conducts and organizes the unique and important functional elements of your mind, into a unified, rhythmic, harmonious balance.

Try some of these tips and let belief play a central role in establishing and maintaining your balance for life. Then you will have a clear sense of how to live in balance.

1. Talk to God. Talk to your personal God, whether you are religious or not. Develop an internal dialog with an entity that represents something you believe in. It could be a religious God who guides you in the principles of your religion, or it could be a personal god who represents the ideal way to work in your career. Or it could be the "god" of Alcoholics Anonymous, a higher power to which you give over control in the daily struggle against alcoholism.

   When you talk to God, you are helping your brain to function according to your system of belief. So have a conversation with your God. Use your internal conversation to review the guiding principles of your system of belief.

2. Take pleasure in miracles. Miracles happen every day. Enjoy them. Take pleasure in the way that the miracles of life reinforce your system of belief.

   The sun rises, your children wake up with a

smile, you live your day in good health, a friendly passerby helps you to load groceries in your car. All of these small events are miracles that represent fundamental beliefs—beliefs about nature, about the basic happiness of children, about altruism and goodwill among people. There are miracles everywhere you look. Enjoy them and let an appreciation of miracles strengthen your practice of belief.

3. Make your home a special place. Consider that your home can strengthen your belief. How? You accomplish this by creating a home environment that symbolizes important aspects of who you are. It could be a vase of cut flowers that remind you of your garden; it could be pictures of people you care about; it could be a religious symbol that you hang on the wall; it could be a bookcase filled with your favorite books; or it could be music that brings helpful memories and feelings to mind.

Make sure to arrange your home environment in a pleasing, harmonious way. Set your sight lines so that you can see the symbols of your belief. Find places for activities that evoke a helpful mind-set. Arrange your furniture to create a pleasing aesthetic. Make a few simple changes in your home to strengthen your mind's ability to believe and evoke the feeling of balance in your day-to-day life.

4. Create a story that you believe in. A story about your belief can be a simple statement such as, "In my day-to-day priorities I am a mother first and bookkeeper second." Or your story could be as

complicated as the story that tells of your pathway or recovery from alcoholism. Create a story in words or pictures that illustrates the ways in which your system of belief guides your life. Then actively think about your story when you are trying to figure out how to balance your life.

5. Carry pictures that strengthen your belief. Visual symbols, like pictures, are powerful reminders of your beliefs. Keep a picture with you. For example, pictures of your kids will remind you of your belief in yourself as a parent. Pictures of your favorite getaway place will remind you of your belief in happiness, and peace. Pictures of your pet will remind you of affection. When life is hurried, when you are feeling out of balance, look at these pictures to help you to believe in yourself.

6. Write down your personal code of ethics. Review it when you need a boost. Whatever guides your morals, your ethics and your well-meaning behavior can be written down as a series of statements that serve as a helpful reminder of what to do. It could be the Ten Commandments, or the ethics of your profession, the Twelve Steps of Alcoholics Anonymous, or even a collection of sayings from your parents. Write them down and review your personal code regularly.

7. Identify your groups. Think about what groups of people you naturally feel close to. You need not meet with the group regularly to belong. All that is necessary for this tip to work, is that you identify

with a group of people who share your interests, your values and your beliefs.

Once you identify your groups, then you have a natural mechanism for identifying and strengthening your belief. It happens when you meet with your group, or think about your group. Then you get in touch with the shared values and beliefs. The connection to a group of like-minded people makes this especially powerful.

8. Look for leaders and become a leader. When you are trying to figure out how to balance life or how to handle a difficult situation, then look for a leader to follow. Pick someone who exemplifies your beliefs. You can find them anywhere: in books, on television, at school, at work, at church or in your family. To make this tip especially powerful, once you have learned from a leader, try leading yourself. You could teach Sunday school, or coach soccer, or simply try to teach your kids a new skill. As you do, your belief deepens, you feel more committed, and the strength of your belief helps you to bring balance to your life.

9. Let your rituals lead you to your beliefs. Do you like to cook dinner for your family? Then perhaps you believe in bringing your family together regularly. Do you go to church services or the temple regularly? Then perhaps you believe in God. Not to trivialize this discussion but, do you brush your teeth every day? Then perhaps you believe that dental hygiene will help to keep your teeth healthy.

Look for your rituals. They can tell you a lot about your beliefs.

10. Honor your ancestors. Since the wisdom of belief is often passed down from the older members of a generation to the young, honoring your ancestors can help you to recognize and strengthen your beliefs. Talk about your ancestors. What did they do? How did they make their way in life? What does the story of their lives have to tell you that is helpful? Visit their gravesites and the places where they lived. By honoring your ancestors you naturally balance the frenetic pace of today's life with a healthy remembrance of time-honored patterns of belief.

An Image of Balance

Seven systems of natural balance: Rules for living to guide you to balance. Each rule derived from the workings of your brain, derived from the workings of your mind, derived from your seven biologic systems of balance; guiding you to a flowing rhythm of energy and thought. Balance.

Here is an image of balance that works for me. As a boy, I loved the ocean. Hour upon hour, with a blue plastic face mask, peering through the sunlit depths to the sandy bottom, looking at the mysteries of clam shells, seaweed, odd pebbles and crabs; buoyant in the warm, salty ocean, I bobbed up and down with the rhythm of the waves. Peaceful. Happy. In balance, as only a child can be.

What is your image of balance? How do you picture

yourself when you are in a flowing rhythm, filled with the joy and pleasure that is the special gift of balanced living?

I cherish that memory of the ocean from my childhood. It captures the feeling of balance, and, like my father's guiding hand, showing me how to skate; like the spiritual resonance of the choir music in my church; like the profound advice of my professional mentors; like my daughter's delicious smile, missing two teeth, happy to see me at the end of my day; the sense I make of these memories is balance. I believe in these memories, these images, these people. They guide me. When, in the course of another busy day, I begin to feel rushed; when I begin to react; when I start to lose myself in the excitement of the day; then I reflect on the images that capture my personal principles, my guiding rules for balance.

Use the ideas, tips and techniques in this book to build your rules for living; to build a program of balance. Let the natural rules of your nervous system lead you to balance. It has worked for me. Time and again I have overcome problems of balance, straightened out my life by applying the rules of balance.

You can, too. Let the natural rules of your body and your mind, rules that have guided our behavior for hundreds of thousands of years, calm you, guide you and lead you to balance. Keep an open mind and you will see. It is not too much more difficult than bobbing in the waves, warmed by the sun, with your blue plastic mask on so that you can see, in a gentle and flowing rhythm, the circumstances of your life.

ABOUT THE AUTHOR

Paul J. Sorgi, M.D., is a psychiatrist practicing in Sudbury, Massachusetts. He is a founding director of The Hallowell Center for Cognitive and Emotional Health, a practice specializing in the evaluation and treatment of depression, anxiety, attention problems and learning problems in children and adults. He attended Tufts University Medical School where he graduated as a member of the Alpha Omega Alpha National Honor Medical Society. Dr. Sorgi trained in psychiatry at the Harvard Medical School. He is currently on the faculty of Harvard Medical School and a consulting physician at McLean Hospital.

Dr. Sorgi has written many professional publications on a variety of topics. He has spoken hundreds of times before local and national audiences on the topics of depression, impulse problems and attention deficit disorder. With Dr. Edward Hallowell, he writes a national, monthly, personal growth and wellness newsletter called *Mind Matters.*

Dr. Sorgi lives in Massachusetts with his two children, Nora and Jack.

Dr. Sorgi can be reached by phone at 978-287-0810, or by e-mail at *pjsorgi@aol.com*.

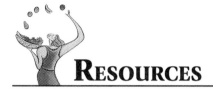

RESOURCES

Chapter One

1. Buss, David. *American Psychologist.* January, 2000. The Evolution of Happiness.
2. Gleick, James. *Faster.* Pantheon Books. New York. 1999
3. Diamond, Jared. *Guns, Germs, and Steel. The Fates of Human Societies.* W.W. Norton & Co. New York. 1998
4. Notzon, Francis C; Komarov, Yuri; Ermakov, Sergei; Sempos, Christopher; Marks, James; Sempos, Elena; *Journal of the American Medical Society.* March 11, 1998. Causes of Declining Life Expectancy in Russia
5. Wilson, E.O. *Consilience. The Unity of Knowledge.* Alfred A. Knopf Inc. New York. 1998
6. Ratey, John J; *Neuropsychiatry of Personality Disorders.* Blackwell Science, Cambridge Ma. 1995
7. Klar, Howard; Siever, Larry J; *Biologic Response Styles.* American Psychiatric Press. Washington, D.C. 1985

Chapter Two

1. Curtis, Brian, A.; Jacobsen, Stanley; Marcus, Elliot, M.; *An Introduction to the Neurosciences.* W.B. Saunders. Philadelphia, Pa. 1972

2. Mesulam, M-Marsel; *Principles of Behavioral Neurology.* F.A. Davis. Philadelphia, Pa. 1987

3. Donald, Merlin; *Origins of the Modern Mind. Three Stages in the Evolution of Culture and Cognition.* Harvard University Press. Cambridge, Ma. 1991

4. Carlson, Neil, R.: *Physiology of Behavior.* Allyn and Bacon. Needham Heights, Ma. 1994

5. Cooper, Jack, R.; Bloom, Floyd, E.; Roth, Robert, H.; *The Biochemical Basis of Neuropharmacology.* Oxford University Press. New York. 1978

6. Lorenz, Konrad; *On Aggression.* Bantam Books. New York. 1971

7. Tarnas, Richard; *The Passion of the Western Mind: Understanding the Ideas That Have Shaped Our World View.* Ballantine Books. New York. 1993

Chapter Three

1. Hallowell, Edward, M. *Connect.* Pantheon Books, New York. 1999

2. Schor, Juliet, B.; *The Overworked American.* Basic Books. New York. 1993

3. Hymowitz, Carol. *The Wall Street Journal.* "In the Lead. Flooded With E-Mail?"

4. Jeffrey, Nancy Ann; *The Wall Street Journal.* Friday May 12, 2000. "A Rude Awakening."

5. Rothbaum Fred; Weisz, John; Pott, Martha; Miyake, Kazuo; Morelli, Gilda; *American Psychologist;* October 2000. "Attachment and Culture."

6. Myers, David, G.; *American Psychologist.* January 2000. "The Funds, Friends, and Faith of Happy People."

7. Lucas, Richard, E.; *Journal of Personality and Social Psychology.* September 6, 2000. "Sensitivity to Rewards May Distinguish Extraverts From Introverts."

8. Deater-Deckard, Kirby; Pickering, Kevin; Dunn, Judith, F.; Golding, Jean; *American Journal of Psychiatry.* June 1998. "Family Structure and Depressive Symptoms in Men Preceding and Following the Birth of a Child."

9. Bowlby, J; *Attachment.* Basic Books: New York. 1969

10. Winnicot, D.W. *The Maturational Process and the Facilitating Environment.* International Universities Press. New York. 1965

11. Kraut, Robert; Patterson, Michael; Lundmark, Vicki; Kiesler, Sara; Mukopadhyay, Tridas; Scherlis, William; *American Psychologist:* September, 1998. "Internet Paradox. A Social Technology That Reduces Social Involvement and Psychological Well-Being?"

12. Goleman, Daniel; *Emotional Intelligence.* Bantam Books. New York: 1997

13. Gardner, Howard; *Multiple Intelligences: The Theory in Practice.* Basic Books. New York: 1993.

Chapter Four

1. Groopman, Jerome. *The New Yorker.* November 13, 2000. Hurting All Over.

2. Feldenkrais, Moshe. *Awareness Through Movement.* HarperCollins Publishers Inc. New York. 1977.

3. Rosenbaum, David, A.; Collyer, Charles, E. *Timing of Behavior.* The MIT Press. Cambridge, Ma. 1998

4. Wilson, Frank, R.; *The Hand. How its Use Shapes the Brain, Language and Human Culture.* Pantheon Books. New York. 1998

5. Fillingham, Roger, B.; Blumenthal, James, A.; *The Use of Aerobic Exercise as a Method of Stress Management.* In Lehrer, Paul, M.; Woolfolk, Robert, L.; *Principles and Practice of Stress Management.* The Guilford Press. New York. 1993

6. Louis, Meera; *The Wall Street Journal.* May 1, 2000. page R7. "Health and Fitness."

7. Jasch, Mary; *The Boston Globe.* November 23, 2000. page A17. "Child Speech Therapy, on Horseback."

8. Shannahoff-Khalsa, David, S.; Ray, Leslie, E.; Levine, Saul; Gallen, Christopher, C. Schwartz, Barry, J.; Sidorowich, John, J.; CNS Spectrums. December 1999. Randomized Controlled Trial of Yogic Meditation Techniques for Patients With Obsessive-Compulsive Disorder.

9. Broocks, Andreas; Bandelow, Borwin; Pekrun, Gunda; George, Annette; Meyer, Tim; Bartmann, Uwe; Hillmer-Vogel, Ursula; Ruther, Eckart; *American Journal of Psychiatry.* May 1998.

Comparison of Aerobic Exercise, Clomipramine, and Placebo in the Treatment of Panic Disorder.

10. Kramer, A.F.; *Nature*. July 29, 2000. "Aging, Fitness and Neurocognitive Function."
11. Dowling, Claudia Glenn; *People Magazine*. January 15, 2001. "Horse Medicine."
12. Maranto, Cheryl, Dileo; Music Therapy and Stress Management. In Lehrer, Paul, M.; Woolfolk, Robert, L.; *Principles and Practice of Stress Management*. The Guilford Press. New York. 1993
13. EMDR: A Promising New Therapy for Trauma and Anxiety. *Mind Matters Newsletter*. October 1998. Mind Matters LLC. 754 Mass. Ave. Arlington, Ma.

Chapter Five

1. Shenk, David; *Data Smog. Surviving the Information Glut.* HarperCollins Publishers Inc. New York. 1997
2. Black, Donald, W.; Belsare, Geeta; Schlosser, Steven; *Journal of Clinical Psychiatry*. December 1999. Clinical Features, Psychiatric Comorbidity, and Heath-Related Quality of Life in Persons Reporting Compulsive Computer Use Behavior.
3. Vaillant, George, E.; *Adaptation to Life. How the Best and the Brightest Came of Age*. Little, Brown and Company. Boston Ma. 1977
4. Piaget, Jean. *Structuralism*. Basic Books: New York. 1970
5. Kimura, Doreen; *Sex and Cognition*. The MIT Press. Cambridge Ma. 1999
6. Horowitz, Mardi; Marmar, Charles; Krupnick, Janice; Wilner, Nancy; Kaltreider, Nancy; Wallerstein, Robert; *Personality Styles and Brief Psychotherapy*. Basic Books, Inc. New York. 1984
7. Klerman, Gerald, L.; Weissman, Myrna, M.; Rounsaville, Bruce, J. Chevron, Eve, S.; *Interpersonal Psychotherapy of Depression*. Basic Books Inc. New York. 1984
8. Beck, A.T.; Rush A.J.; Shaw, B.F.; Emery, G.; *Cognitive Therapy of Depression*. Guilford Press: New York. 1979
9. Kileen, Wendy. *The Boston Sunday Globe*. April 23, 2000.

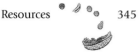

Healing Arts. The Lynn Raw Art Works brings the tools of creativity to people who need more than talk.

10. Lubinski, David; Benbow, Camilla Persson; *American Psychologist*. January 2000. States of Excellence.

Chapter Six

1. Sullivan, Allanna. *The Wall Street Journal*. Monday May 1, 2000. Health and Medicine. To understand why Americans eat so poorly these days keep this in mind: So little time, so much money.

2. Winslow, Ron. *The Wall Street Journal*. Monday May 1, 2000. Health and Medicine. Why Fitness Matters. An Imbalance between our genetic makeup and modern society leaves us vulnerable to all sorts of diseases.

3. Knapp, Caroline. *Drinking: A Love Story*. Dell Publishing Group Inc. New York. 1996

4. Hingson, Ralph. W.; Heeren, Timothy; Jamanka, Amber; Howland, Jonathan; *Journal of the American Medical Association*. September 27, 2000. "Age of Drinking Onset and Unintentional Injury Involvement After Drinking."

5. Toomey, Kathleen, E.; Rothenberg, Richard, B.; *Journal of the American Medical Association*. July 26, 2000. "Sex and Cyberspace-Virtual Networks Leading to High-Risk Sex."

6. Klausner, Jeffrey, D.; Wolf, Wendy; Fisher-Ponce, Lyn; Zolt, Ilene; Katz, Mitchell, H.; *Journal of the American Medical Association*. July 26, 2000. "Tracing a Syphilis Outbreak Through Cyberspace."

7. Pinel, John, P.J.; Assanand, Sunaina; Lehman, Darrin, R.; *American Psychologist*. October 2000: "Hunger, Eating and Ill Health."

8. Victoroff, Jeff; *Psychiatric Times*. February, 1999: "Why We Are Fat."

9. Wolpe, Joseph; *The Practice of Behavior Therapy*. Pergamon Press Inc. Elmsford, New York. 1973

10. Womble, Leslie. G.; Wang, Shirley, S.; Wadden, Thomas, A.; *The Economics of Neuroscience*. August 2000. Behavioral Treatment of Obesity.

11. Devlin, Michael, J.; Yanovski, Susan, Z.; Wilson, Terence, G.; *American Journal of Psychiatry*. June 2000: Obesity: What Mental Health Professionals Need to Know.
12. Carnes, Patrick, J.; *CNS Spectrums*. October 2000: Sexual Addiction and Compulsion: Recognition, Treatment, and Recovery.
13. Agras, W. Stewart; Walsh, Timothy; Fairburn, Christopher; Wilson, Terence, G.; Kraemer, Helena, C.; *Archives of General Psychiatry*. May 2000: A Multicenter Comparison of Cognitive-Behavioral Therapy and Interpersonal Psychotherapy for Bulimia Nervosa.

Chapter Seven

1. Vail, Priscilla; *Emotion: The On/Off Switch for Learning*. Modern Learning Press. Rosemont, NJ. 1994
2. Damasio, Antonio, R.; Descartes' Error: Emotion, Reason, and the Human Brain. Avon Books. New York. 1994
3. Maggini, Carlo; *CNS Spectrums*. August 2000: Psychobiology of Boredom
4. Johnson, Debra, L.; Wiebe, John, S.; Gold, Sherri, M.; Andreasen, Nancy, C.; Hichwa, Richard, D.; Watkins, Leonard, G.; Ponto, Laura L. Boles; *American Journal of Psychiatry*. February, 1999: Cerebral Blood Flow and Personality: A Positron Emission Tomography Study.
5. Koepp, M.J. et al; Nature. May 1998. Evidence of Striatal Dopamine Release During a Video Game.
6. Richards, Jane, M.; Gross, James, J.; *Journal of Personality and Social Psychology*. September 6, 2000. Strategies for Regulating Emotions Affect Memory.
7. Cyranowski, Jill, M; Frank, Ellen; Young, Elizabeth; Shear, Katherine; *Archives of General Psychiatry*. January 2000: Adolescent Onset of the Gender Difference in Lifetime Rates of Major Depression.
8. Silberg, Judy; Pickles, Andrew; Rutter, Micheal; Hewitt, John; Simonoff, Emily; Maes, Hermine; Carbonneau, Rene; Murrelle, Lenn; Foley, Debra; Eaves, Linden; *Archives of General Psychiatry*.

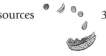

March 1999. The Influence of Genetic Factors and Life Stress on Depression Among Adolescent Girls.

9. Kornblut, Anne, E. *The Boston Globe*. May 6, 2000. Bigger, faster coasters tied to head injuries. Findings in new study alarming, doctors say.

10. Costello, Daniel. *The Wall Street Journal*. January 16, 2001. Incidents of "Desk Rage" Disrupt America's Offices.

11. Trottman, Melanie; Cummins, Chip; *The Wall Street Journal*. September 26, 2000. Passenger's Death Prompts Calls for Improved "Air Rage" Procedures.

12. Weber, Thomas, E.; *The Wall Street Journal*. September 25, 2000. "Worried Your E-Mail May Offend the Boss? Just Check It for Chilis."

13. Simonton, Dean, Keith; *American Psychologist*. January 2000. Creativity: Cognitive, Personal, Developmental and Social Aspect.

14. Waldman, Peter. *The Wall Street Journal*. May 12, 2000. A Tragedy Transforms a Right-Handed Artist Into a Lefty-and a Star.

15. Erikson, Erik, H.; *Childhood and Society*. W.W. Norton and Co. New York. 1963

16. Burns, David, D.; *Feeling Good: The New Mood Therapy*. Signet. New York. 1980

Chapter Eight

1. Hobson, J. Allan; *The Chemistry of Conscious States: How the Brain Changes Its Mind*. Little, Brown and Company. Boston, Ma. 1994

2. Hauri, Peter; Orr, Peter, C.; *The Sleep Disorders*. in Current Concepts. The Upjohn Company (now Pharmacia/Upjohn). Kalamazoo, Mi. 1982

3. Pigeau, R.; Naitoh, P.; Buguet, A.; McCann, C.; Baranski, J.; Taylor, M.; Thompson, M.; Mack, I.; *Journal of Sleep Research*. 1995: 4, (212-228) Modafinil, d-amphetamine and placebo during 64 hours of sustained mental work. I. Effects on mood, fatigue, cognitive performance and body temperature.

4. Allen, Richard, P; *Sleep Medicine* 1 2000: 149-150. Article Reviewed: Impact of sleep debt on metabolic and endocrine function.

5. Shellenbarger, Sue. *The Wall Street Journal*. September 20, 2000. Some Employers Begin to Find What Helps Shiftworker Families.

6. Lyznicki, James, M.; Doege, Theodore, C.; Davis, Ronald, M; Williams, Michael, A; *Journal of the American Medical Association*. June 17, 1998. "Sleepiness, Driving and Motor Vehicle Crashes."

7. Johnson, Eric, O.; Roehrs, Timothy; Roth, Thomas; Breslau, Naomi; *Sleep*. Volume 22, Number 4, 1999. "Epidemiology of Medication as Aids to Alertness in Early Adulthood."

8. Rosenthal, Norman, E; Blehar, Mary, C.; *Seasonal Affective Disorders and Phototherapy*. The Guilford Press. New York. 1989

9. Chesson, Andrew, L; Littner, Michael; Davila, David; Anderson, W. MacDowell; Grigg-Damberger, Madeleine; Hartse, Kristyna; Johnson, Stephen; Wise, Merrill; *Sleep*. Volume 22, Number 5, 1999. "Practice Parameters for the Use of Light Therapy in the Treatment of Sleep Disorders."

10. Chesson, Andrew, L.; Anderson, W. MacDowell; Littner, Michael; Davila, David; Hartse, Kristyna; Johnson, Stephen; Wise, Merrill; Rafecas, Jose; *Sleep*. Volume 22, Number 8, 1999. "Practice Parameters for the Nonpharmacologic Treatment of Chronic Insomnia."

11. Dorsey, Cynthia, M.; Teicher, Martin, H.; Cohen-Zion, Mairav; Stefanovic, Louis; Satlin, Andrew; Tartarini, Wendy; Lukas, Scott, E.; *Sleep*. Volume 22, Number 7. 1999 "Core Body Temperature and Sleep of Older Female Insomniacs Before and After Passive Body Heating."

12. Okamoto-Mizuno, Kazue; Mizuno, Koh; Michie, Saeko; Maeda, Akiko; Iizuka, Sachiko; *Sleep*. Volume 22, Number 6, 1999. "Effects of Humid Heat Exposure on Human Sleep Stages and Body Temperature."

Chapter Nine

1. Frank, Jerome, D; *Persuasion and Healing*. The Johns Hopkins University Press. Schocken Books. New York 1974.

2. Gallagher, Winifred; *The Power of Place. How Our Surroundings Shape Our Thoughts, Emotions, and Actions.* HarperCollins Publishers Inc. New York. 1993

3. Hallowell, Edward, M.; *Worry: Controlling It and Using It Wisely.* Pantheon Books. New York. 1997

4. Kaminer, Wendy; *Sleeping With Extra-Terrestrials: The Rise of Irrationalism and Perils of Piety.* Vintage Books, a division of Random House. New York. 2000.

5. Groopman, Jerome; *The New Yorker.* April 10, 2000. "The Doubting Disease."

6. Brier, Bob; *The Murder of Tutankhamen.* Berkley Books. New York. 1998.

7. Himle, Joseph, A.; Abelson, James, J.; Haghightgou, Hedieh; Hill, Elizabeth, M.: Nesse, Randolph, M.; Curtis, George, C.; *American Journal of Psychiatry.* August 1999. "Effect of Alcohol on Phobic Anxiety."

8. Flapan, Deborah; *Medscape Wire/Health Psychology. www.medscape.com.* November 21, 2000. "Life Perspective Can Affect Women's Health."

9. Salovey, Peter; Rothman, Alexander, J.; Detweiler, Jerusha, B.; Steward, Wayne, T.; *American Psychologist.* January 2000. "Emotional States and Physical Health."

10. Lipsitz, Joshua, D.; Markowitz, John, C.; Cherry, Sabrina; Fyer, Abby, J; *American Journal of Psychiatry.* November 1999. "Open Trial of Interpersonal Psychotherapy for the treatment of Social Phobia."

11. Taylor, Shelley, E.; Kemeny, Margaret, E.; Reed, Geoffrey, M.; Bower, Julienne, E.; Gruenewald, Tara, L.; *American Psychologist.* January 2000. "Psychological Resources, Positive Illusions, and Health."

12. Baltes, Paul, B.; Staudinger, Ursula, M.; *American Psychologist.* January 2000. Wisdom: "A Metaheuristic (Pragmatic) to Orchestrate Mind and Virtue Toward Excellence."

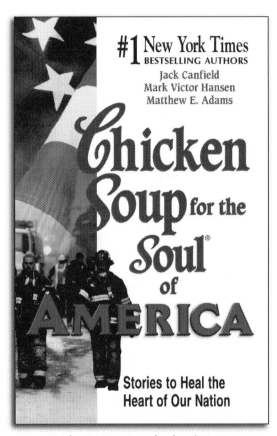

#1 New York Times
BESTSELLING AUTHORS
Jack Canfield
Mark Victor Hansen
Matthew E. Adams

Chicken Soup for the Soul® of AMERICA

**Stories to Heal the
Heart of Our Nation**

Code #0065 • Paperback • $12.95

Celebrating the courage and triumph of the American spirit this book pays tribute to the American hero.

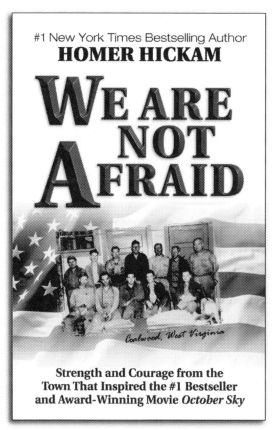

#1 New York Times Bestselling Author
HOMER HICKAM

WE ARE NOT AFRAID

Coalwood, West Virginia

**Strength and Courage from the
Town That Inspired the #1 Bestseller
and Award-Winning Movie *October Sky***

Code #012X • Paperback • $12.95

Fear is a distressing emotion. Hickam provides indispensable steps to help you overcome your fear, both real and imagined, to find courage and strength. This book couldn't be more timely—or more needed—than it is today.

UNLEASH YOUR METABOLISM, LOSE WEIGHT & FEEL GREAT!

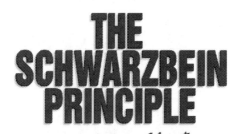

Code #6803 • Paperback • $12.95

Based on sound research and the success of thousands of people, this book proves that excess weight, degenerative disease and accelerated aging can be controlled—and reversed—in a healthful way.